D0471884

MUSCLE &FITNESS

101 GET-LEAN
WORKOUTS AND STRATEGIES

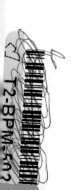

T2-BPM-502

ACKNOWLEDGMENTS

This publication is based on articles written by **John Berardi, Ph.D.; Guillermo Escalante; Jon Finkel; Rob Fitzgerald; Jon Hinds; Myatt Murphy; Sara Polston; Jim Stoppani, Ph.D.; Mark Thorpe; Matt Tuthill; Eric Velazquez;** and **Joe Wuebben**

Cover photography by **Andrew Hetherington**

Photography and illustrations by: **Iconmen.com, Art Brewer, Dylan Coulter, Michael Darter, Bill Diodato, Ian Logan, Robert Reiff, Marc Royce, Ian Spanier, Michael Touna, Larissa Underwood,** and **Pavel Ythjall**

Project editor is **Joe Wuebben**

Project creative director is **Anthony Scerri**

Project copy editor is **Cat Perry**

Project photo assistant is **Amy Wolff**

Founding chairman is **Joe Weider.** Chairman and CEO of American Media, Inc., is **David Pecker.**

©2012, American Media, Inc. All Rights Reserved. No part of this publication may be reproduced or incorporated into any information retrieval system, electronic or mechanical, without the written permission of the copyright owner. Inquiries regarding permission for use of material contained in this publication should be addressed to: American Media, Inc., 4 New York Plaza, New York, NY 10004, Attn: Rights and Permissions.

This book is available in quantity at special discounts for your group or organization. For further information, contact:

Triumph Books
814 N. Franklin Street
Chicago, IL 60610
(312) 337-0747
www.triumphbooks.com
ISBN: 978-1-60078-736-2

Printed in USA.

MUSCLE &F FITNESS
101 GET-LEAN
WORKOUTS AND STRATEGIES

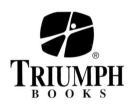

TRIUMPH
BOOKS

TRIUMPHBOOKS.COM

CONTENTS

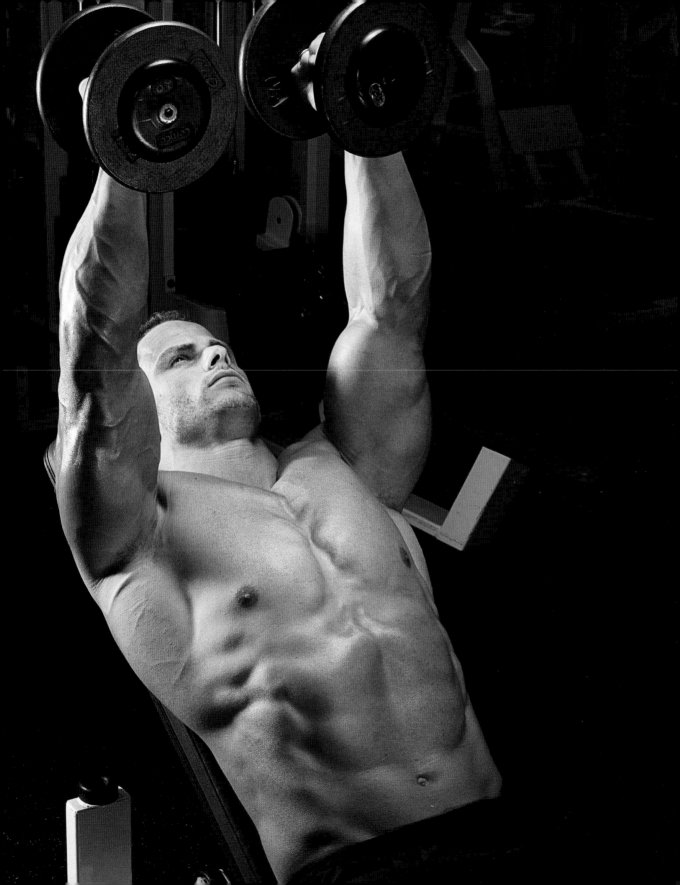

CHAPTER 1

GET RIPPED IN 12 WEEKS

BURN LOADS OF BODY FAT WITH THIS HIGH-INTENSITY TRAINING PROGRAM AND NUTRITION PLAN

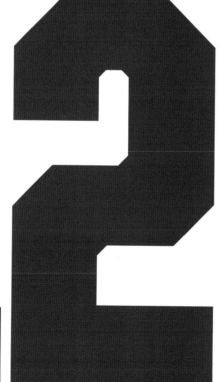

Who says a get-lean phase has to take place at the beginning of the year or heading into summer? Any time is a good time for your abs to be shredded and the rest of your muscles sliced and diced just the same. Which is why the timing is perfect right now for this 12-week fat-burning, weightlifting, and cardio programs and meal plan. The training is high-volume and intense, and the diet manipulates macronutrients in such a way that your metabolism will hit the roof. Three months from now you'll be as lean as ever, if not sooner.

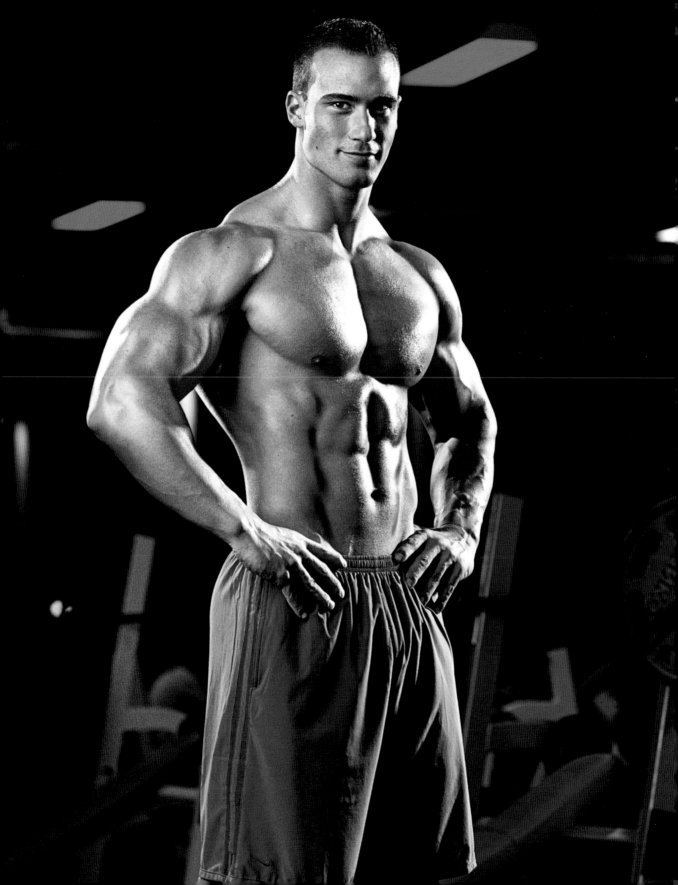

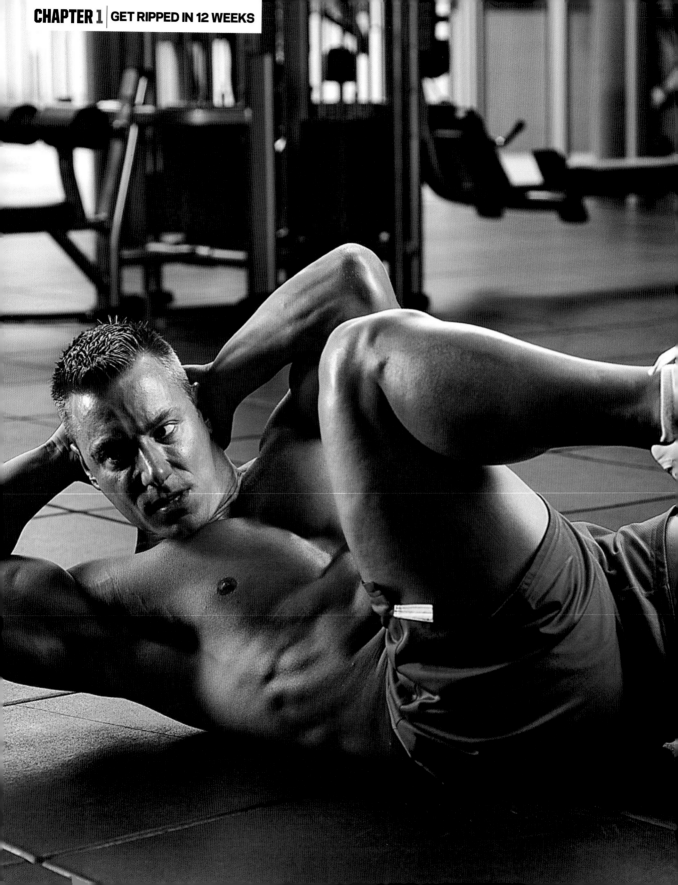

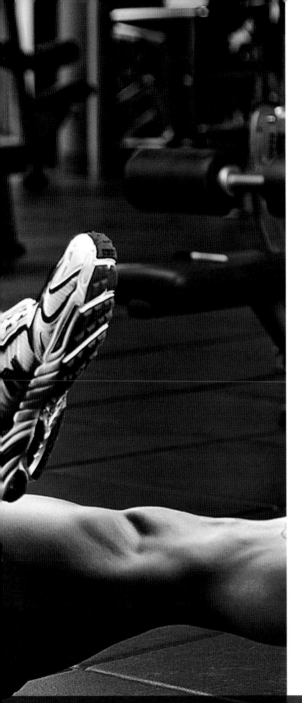

CARDIO CONSIDERATIONS

As with your weight workouts, your approach to cardio will vary each week. You'll alternate between steady-state cardio and high-intensity interval sessions to burn fat through different mechanisms. Each week you'll stride through as many as five cardio workouts, each lasting 20–60 minutes.

You can get more out of these sessions by performing them before breakfast or post-workout; saving cardio for after high-rep sessions with a given body part can help burn more subcutaneous body fat from that area. The fat, which is mobilized through exercise, is then used as fuel during cardio rather than redepositing itself under your skin. With that in mind, try to get your cardio in after your ab workout(s) each week and schedule a few other sessions for first thing in the morning.

SHREDDING SEASON

For the next 12 weeks we give you a full playbook: heavy sets of six reps, moderately weighted sets of 10–12 reps, and lighter sets of 20. For abs, you'll dabble in 30-rep sets at times, giving your belly the opportunity to burn some of the released fat after a hardcore cardio session. As for cardio, let's just say you're going to work hard and sweat through plenty of towels. But as you adapt and improve week after week, your body will switch to calorie-burning autopilot, where each workout will force your body to call upon its stubborn fat stores for energy. By the end of the program, you can expect to be at your absolute leanest.

AIR BIKE CROSSOVER CRUNCH

INTENSELY LEAN

While the exercises laid out in this program aren't too complicated, the offbeat split and gamut of rep ranges will likely take some getting used to. But don't worry, the routine described above and presented on the following pages is structured to help you recruit boatloads of fibers within your targeted muscle groups—and thus burn more fat and grow more muscle—over the next 12 weeks. The addition of cardio will serve only to speed things up.

RIPPED IN 12 WEEKS CARDIO

WEEKS 1, 3, 5
PERFORM FOUR TIMES PER WEEK

EXERCISE	DURATION	INTENSITY (PE[1])
Treadmill Walk	45 min.	5
or Exercise Bike	45 min.	5
or StepMill	45 min.	5

WEEKS 2, 4, 6
PERFORM FOUR TIMES PER WEEK

EXERCISE	DURATION	INTENSITY (PE[1])[2]
Treadmill Run	20 min.	9/2
or Exercise Bike	20 min.	9/2
or StepMill	20 min.	9/2

WEEKS 7, 9, 11
PERFORM FIVE TIMES PER WEEK

EXERCISE	DURATION	INTENSITY (PE[1])
Treadmill Jog	60 min.	5
or Exercise Bike	60 min.	5
or StepMill	60 min.	5

WEEKS 8, 10, 12
PERFORM FIVE TIMES PER WEEK

EXERCISE	DURATION	INTENSITY (PE[1])[2]
Treadmill Run	30 min.	9/2
or Exercise Bike	30 min.	9/2
or StepMill	30 min.	9/2

1 Perceived exertion (PE) is how hard you feel your body is working on a scale of 1 to 10 based on the physical sensations you experience.

2 Perform your cardio interval-style, alternating one-minute bouts of high-intensity sprints with more recuperative stretches of one minute for the time prescribed.

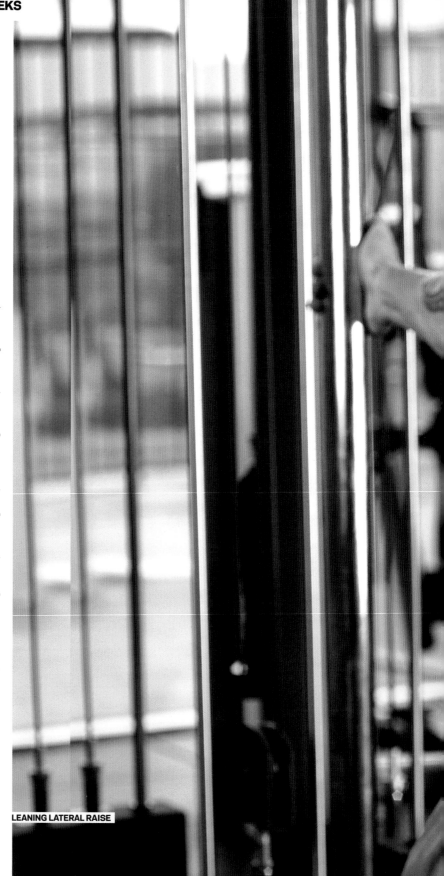

LEANING LATERAL RAISE

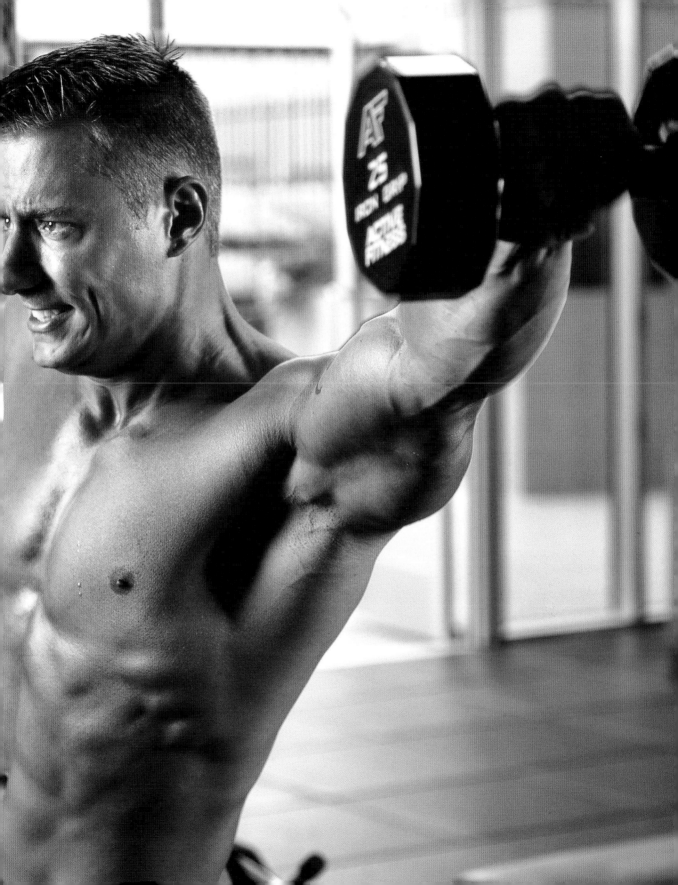

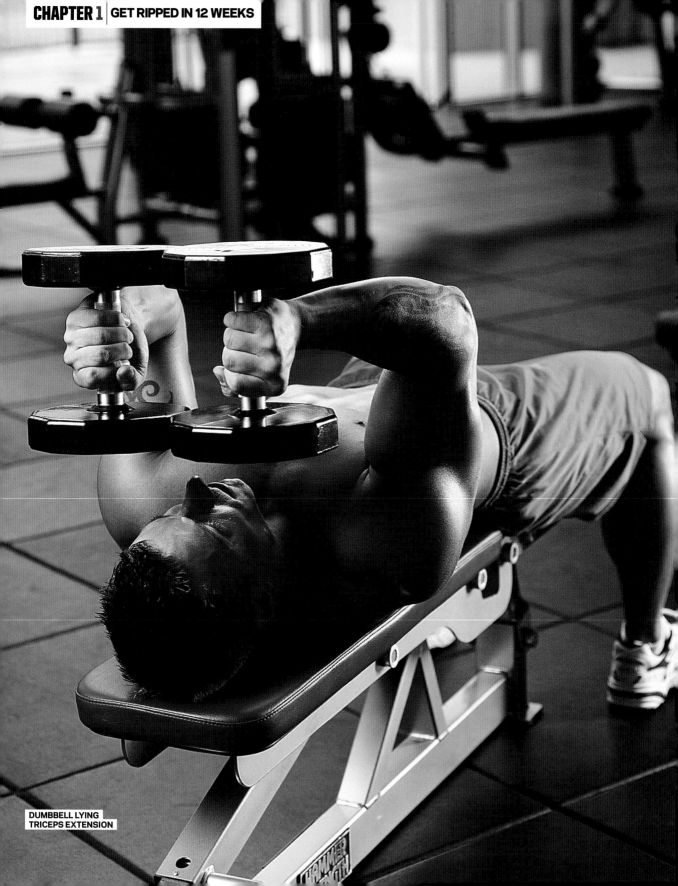

**DUMBBELL LYING
TRICEPS EXTENSION**

TRAINING PROGRAM A

Weeks 1, 3, 5, 7, 9, 11:

During odd-numbered weeks—if we count today as Day 1 of Week 1—you'll train for strength and hypertrophy with low-to-moderate rep ranges. You'll focus on heavy compound lifts, usually with barbells, to get your muscles growing. Shorter rest periods (45-60 seconds) are intended to help maximize your energy stores—studies have shown that most individuals will be adequately recovered after one minute as opposed to three—while keeping your heart rate up for added metabolic benefits.

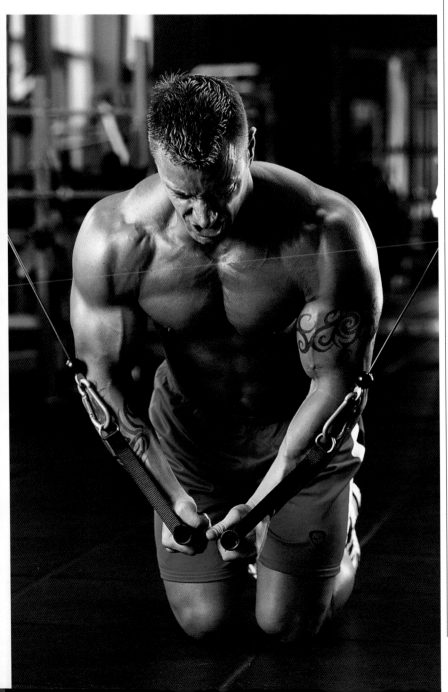

WEEKS 1, 3, 5, 7, 9, 11
DAY 1 | SHOULDERS + TRAPS + ABS

EXERCISE	SETS	REPS
Barbell Overhead Press	5	6,6,10,10,12
Leaning Lateral Raise	5	6,6,10,10,12
Upright Row	5	6,6,10,10,12
Bentover Lateral Raise	5	6,6,10,10,12
Barbell Shrug	5	6,6,10,10,12
Weighted Crunch	3	10,10,20
Air Bike Crossover Crunch	3	10,10,20

DAY 2 | TRICEPS + BICEPS

EXERCISE	SETS	REPS
Dumbbell Lying Triceps Extension	5	6,6,10,10,12
Pushdown	5	6,6,10,10,12
Dumbbell Overhead Triceps Extension	5	6,6,10,10,12
Barbell Curl	5	6,6,10,10,12
Dumbbell Incline Curl	5	6,6,10,10,12
Preacher Curl	5	6,6,10,10,12

DAY 3 | LEGS

EXERCISE	SETS	REPS
Squat	5	6,6,10,10,12
Leg Press	5	6,6,10,10,12
Leg Extension	5	6,6,10,10,12
Lunge	5	6,6,10,10,12
Romanian Deadlift	5	6,6,10,10,12
Lying Leg Curl	5	6,6,10,10,12
Standing Calf Raise	2	12
Seated Calf Raise	2	12
Donkey Calf Raise	2	12

DAY 5 | CHEST + ABS

EXERCISE	SETS	REPS
Bench Press	5	6,6,10,10,12
Incline Bench Press	5	6,6,10,10,12
Decline Bench Press	5	6,6,10,10,12
Weighted Dip	5	6,6,10,10,12
Kneeling Cable Crossover	5	6,6,10,10,12
Weighted Crunch	3	10,10,20
Reverse Crunch	3	10,10,20

DAY 6 | BACK

EXERCISE	SETS	REPS
Deadlift	5	6,6,10,10,12
Barbell Row	5	6,6,10,10,12
T-bar Row	5	6,6,10,10,12
Seated Cable Row	5	6,6,10,10,12
Wide-grip Lat Pulldown	5	6,6,10,10,12

KNEELING CABLE CROSSOVER

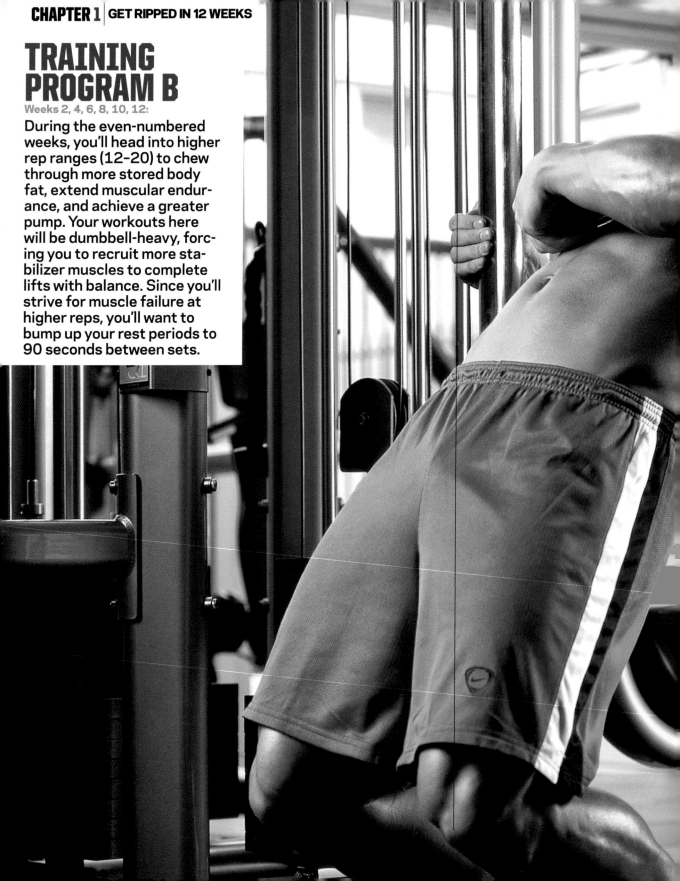

TRAINING PROGRAM B

Weeks 2, 4, 6, 8, 10, 12:

During the even-numbered weeks, you'll head into higher rep ranges (12–20) to chew through more stored body fat, extend muscular endurance, and achieve a greater pump. Your workouts here will be dumbbell-heavy, forcing you to recruit more stabilizer muscles to complete lifts with balance. Since you'll strive for muscle failure at higher reps, you'll want to bump up your rest periods to 90 seconds between sets.

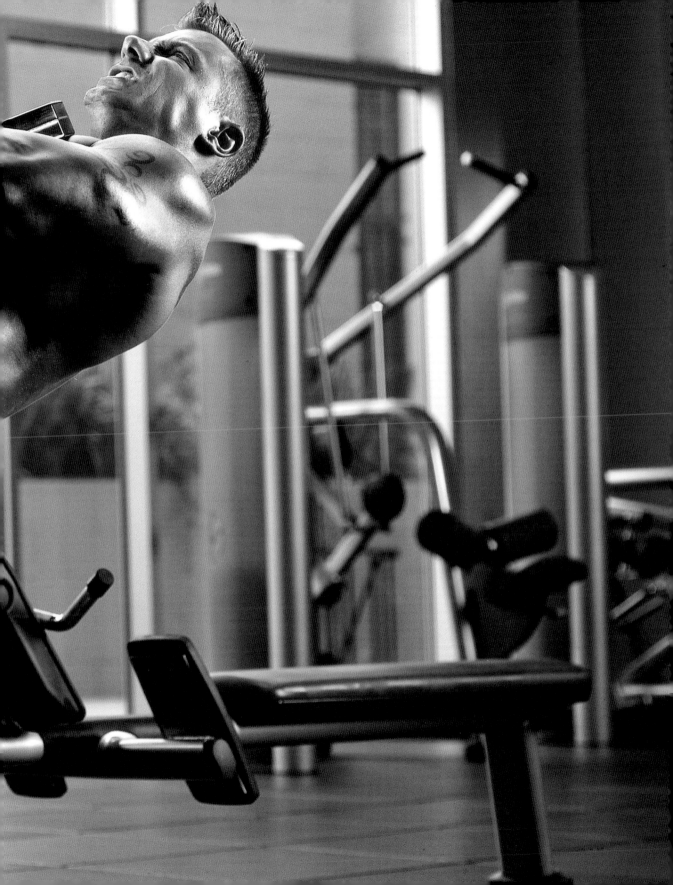

GET RIPPED NUTRTION

MAXIMIZE FAT-BURNING WITH THIS GET-LEAN MEAL PLAN THAT COMPLEMENTS OUR 12-WEEK TRAINING PROGRAM

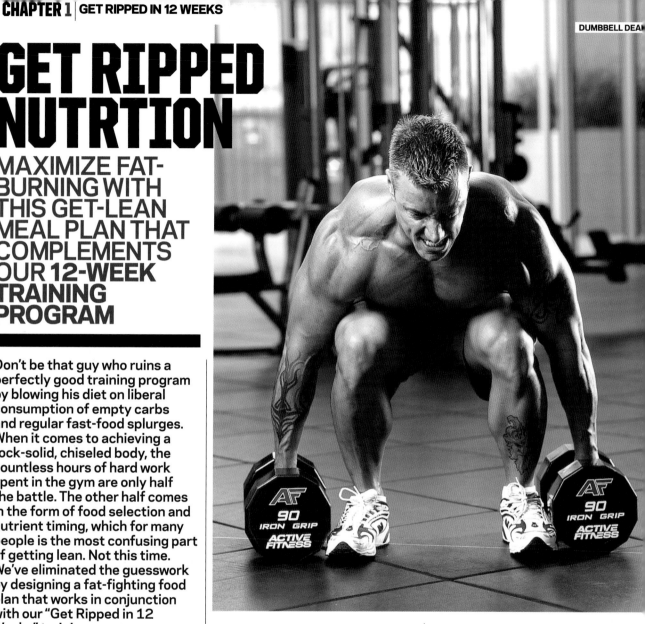

DUMBBELL DEA▮

Don't be that guy who ruins a perfectly good training program by blowing his diet on liberal consumption of empty carbs and regular fast-food splurges. When it comes to achieving a rock-solid, chiseled body, the countless hours of hard work spent in the gym are only half the battle. The other half comes in the form of food selection and nutrient timing, which for many people is the most confusing part of getting lean. Not this time. We've eliminated the guesswork by designing a fat-fighting food plan that works in conjunction with our "Get Ripped in 12 Weeks" training program.

The following meals provide about 14 calories per pound of body weight per day, which is about 2,500 calories for a 180-pound guy. Throughout the 12 weeks, protein intake will remain high to jump-start your metabolism and preserve lean mass. Each week aim to get 1–1.5 grams of protein per pound of body weight, or 180–270 grams per day for the 180-pounder.

Carb intake will vary depending on each week's training goal. During the weeks you follow Training Program A (emphasis on strength and size), shoot for 1.25 grams of carbs per pound per day (225 grams) to supply the energy muscles need. When following Training Program B (emphasis on muscle endurance and fat burning), reduce carbs to 0.75 gram per pound (135 grams per day) to encourage your body to use body fat stores for energy.

As for dietary fat, intake will be 0.4–0.5 gram per pound (70–90 grams per day), accounting for 25%–30% of total daily calories. You'll notice during Program B that when carbs are lower, fat and protein intakes increase to provide the calories needed to help maintain lean muscle mass. Eating healthy omega-3s and monounsaturated fats will remain a priority to further enhance fat-burning and aid your recovery process.

SAMPLE MEAL PLAN PROGRAM A

Breakfast
1 whole-wheat English muffin
2 eggs + 4 egg whites
1 slice low-fat cheese

Midmorning Snack
1 cup low-fat Greek yogurt
1 cup pineapple

Lunch
Fajitas:
6 oz top sirloin
2 whole-wheat Mission Carb Balance Tortilla (6" diameter)
1 cup bell pepper
1 cup lettuce
1/4 cup onion

Pre-workout
1 scoop whey protein
1 apple

Post-workout
1 scoop whey protein
2 cups low-fat milk

Dinner
8 oz pork tenderloin
1 cup quinoa
1 cup broccoli

Bedtime Snack
1 scoop casein protein
1 tbsp flaxseed oil

DAILY TOTALS
2,505 calories
261g protein
201g carbs
73g fat
39g fiber
2,839 mg sodium

SAMPLE MEAL PLAN PROGRAM B

Breakfast
1 scoop whey protein
1 cup low-fat Greek yogurt
1 cup strawberries
2 tbsp ground flaxseeds

Midmorning Snack
2 string cheese sticks
10 whole-wheat crackers

Lunch
6 oz roast beef
2 cups mixed green salad
½ cup tomato
½ cup cucumber
2 tbsp sunflower seeds
2 tbsp olive oil/vinegar dressing

Pre-workout
1 scoop whey protein
6 multigrain rice cakes

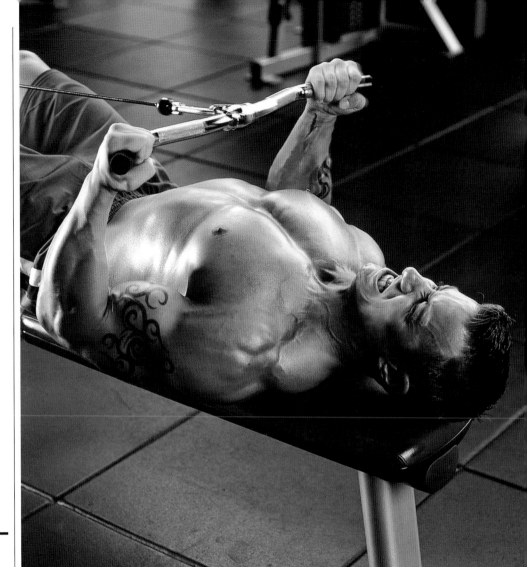

LYING CABLE CURL

Post-workout
8 oz chicken breast
1 medium white potato

Dinner
9 oz tilapia
2 cups green beans

Bedtime Snack
1 scoop casein protein
1 oz mixed nuts

DAILY TOTALS
2,462 calories
283g protein
139g carbs
86g fat
30g fiber
2,239mg sodium

SAMPLE REST DAY MEALS

Breakfast
1 whole-wheat Mission Carb Balance Tortilla (6" diameter)
3 eggs
½ cup bell pepper
1/4 cup onion
1 cup spinach

Midmorning Snack
1 scoop whey protein
1 orange

Lunch
8 oz chicken breast
1 cup brown rice

Mid-afternoon Snack
8 oz salmon
2 cups broccoli

1/3 cup hummus

Dinner
8 oz flank steak
2 cups zucchini

Bedtime Snack
1 cup low-fat cottage cheese
1 tbsp flaxseed oil

DAILY TOTALS
2,351 calories
257g protein
126g carbs
91g fat
26g fiber
2,393mg sodium

Note: Mix protein powders according to label directions.

CHAPTER 2

SCULPT YOUR MIDSECTION IN JUST SIX WEEKS WITH THIS HARD-HITTING TRAINING PROGRAM

SIX-PACK SOLUTION

THE NEXT TIME you stumble upon that Sunday-morning infomercial touting an ab-training gadget as the solution to the perfect six-pack, change the channel. Watch *SportsCenter*, *Meet the Press*, or even *Baywatch* reruns—anything but a $99 glorified crunch that claims to melt flab from your midsection. No one thing alone will get you a six-pack; it takes a multipronged approach of weight training, isolated ab work, intense cardio, and a clean diet. Even though it won't happen overnight, our six-week plan will reveal an impressive set of abs when followed diligently. Its basic parameters are similar to the program in Chapter 1, only with more emphasis placed on the midsection and a tighter deadline. But this plan—unlike the aforementioned infomercial—is about more than just a bunch of ab exercises. You can't get a shredded midsection without ramping up your metabolism, and you can't ramp up your metabolism without hitting the gym hard with a full-body program.

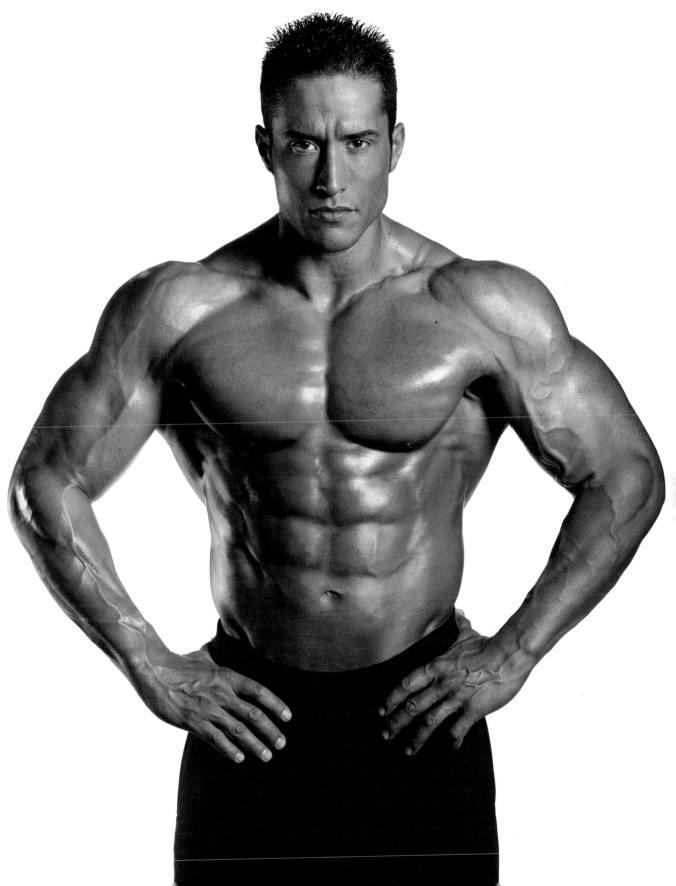

HEAVY LIFTING

PLATEHEAD DECLINE SITUP
START: Lie faceup on a decline situp board, or decline bench with your feet secured under the rollers, holding a light weight plate just above your forehead. (Start with a 10-pound plate and progress to a 25-pounder.)
EXECUTION: Contract your abs to initiate a full situp, keeping the plate on your head throughout. Slowly return to the start position.

LIFTING WEIGHTS seems to be the missing link in most people's efforts to get six-pack abs. Talk to the average guy with this goal in mind and he'll probably tell you about all the cardio he's doing in the gym. Ask him if he's hitting the weights hard and he'll likely respond, "No, I'm not trying to get big, I just want to be defined." (Feel free to roll your eyes at this point, or even punch him.)

"When people throw the word *lean* around, what most of them forget is *lean* means lean body mass, which is muscle," says Jesse Burdick, C.S.C.S., owner and founder of Prevail Fitness in Pleasanton, CA, and a trainer at Re-Active Gym. "Just doing cardio isn't enough to get a six-pack. The more of a full-body weight-training workout you do, the more lean mass you'll have and the higher your metabolism will be. These are synergistic in helping you achieve a six-pack."

In other words, a sound lifting program is key to shedding body fat around the midsection and everywhere else on the body. That's why the following routine entails six days a week of hardcore weightlifting, broken into a body-part split in which you train each major muscle group twice weekly. If the goal of the program were strictly hypertrophy with less emphasis on getting lean, training each body part just once each week might suffice. But boosting metabolism and burning calories are top priorities here, so training frequency is high.

Big exercises take precedence in the program for one simple reason: They work more muscles and, as a result, increase the metabolism that much more. "Multijoint exercises are the kings of muscle recruitment," Burdick says. "Why would you want to recruit just one muscle group when you can force your whole body to work? With big multijoint moves you'll add lean mass quicker, which goes back to that synergistic effect: The more muscle you use, the higher your body mass and metabolism."

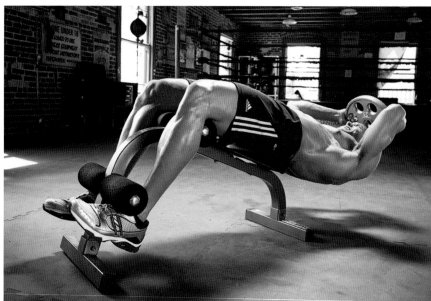

The rep ranges in the program vary from low to high. With bench presses, deadlifts, and squats you'll employ heavy sets of five reps to build strength and stimulate the central nervous system, followed by another five sets of 10 reps in Weeks 1–3 to promote hypertrophy through the use of moderate reps and high volume. Reps on assistance exercises typically fall in the 12–20 range; again, boosting your metabolism through muscle growth is the primary rationale here.

Coupled with mostly moderate-rep ranges are short rest periods designed to maximize fat loss. The majority of breaks are 45–60 seconds, except on arm days, when that decreases to 30 seconds. Even on benches, deads, and squats, rest is fairly brief at 90 seconds tops.

TRAINING SPLIT

DAY	WORKOUT	
	A.M.	P.M.
Monday	Cardio: "High"	Weights: Legs, Abs
Tuesday	Weights: Chest, Back, Abs	Cardio: "Moderate"
Wednesday	Cardio: "Low"	Weights: Triceps, Biceps, Delts, Abs
Thursday	Cardio: "High"	Weights: Posterior Chain, Abs
Friday	Weights: Chest, Back, Abs	Cardio: "Moderate"
Saturday	Cardio: "Low"	Weights: Triceps, Biceps, Delts, Abs
Sunday	Off	Off

For cardio routines, see "Burning Down the House" on page 30.

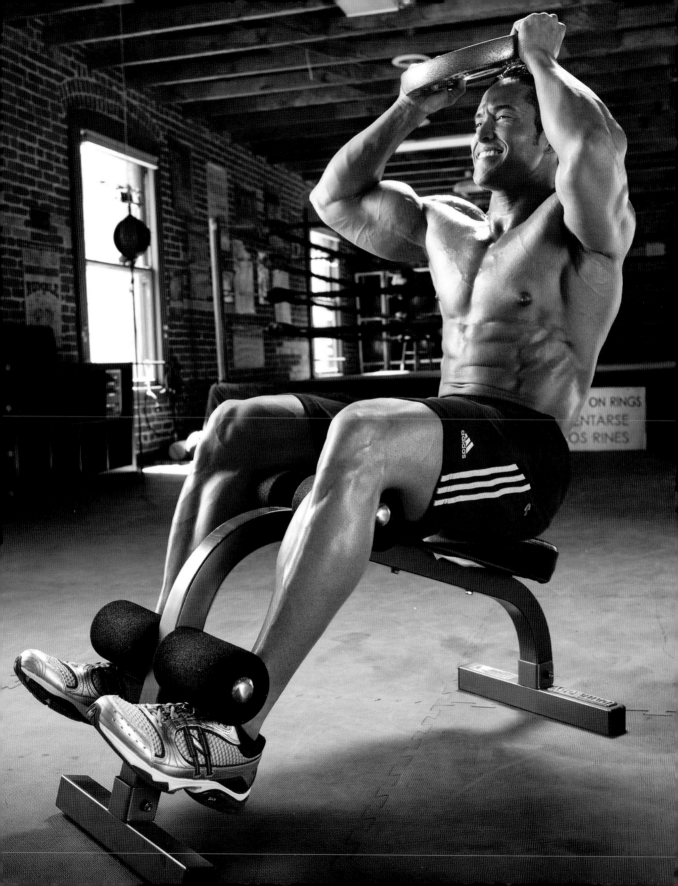

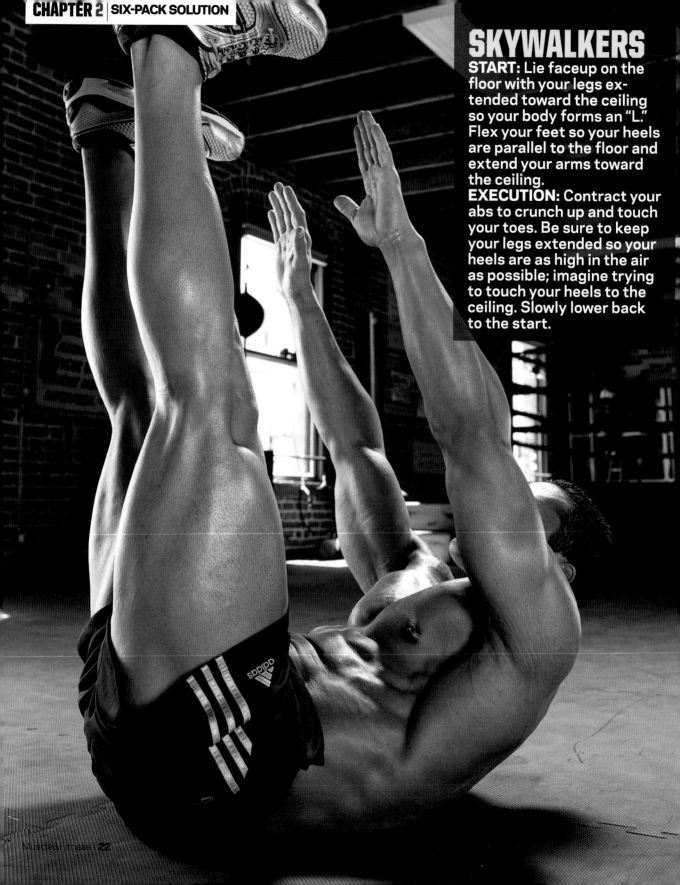

SKYWALKERS

START: Lie faceup on the floor with your legs extended toward the ceiling so your body forms an "L." Flex your feet so your heels are parallel to the floor and extend your arms toward the ceiling.

EXECUTION: Contract your abs to crunch up and touch your toes. Be sure to keep your legs extended so your heels are as high in the air as possible; imagine trying to touch your heels to the ceiling. Slowly lower back to the start.

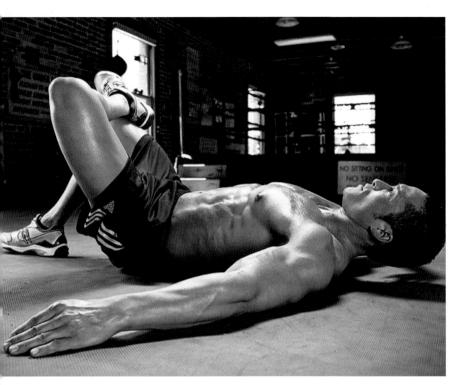

FIGURE-4 CRUNCH

START: Lie faceup on the floor with your knees bent and feet flat. Cross your left leg over so your left ankle rests on your right knee. Place your right hand behind your head with your elbow pointing out to the side.
EXECUTION: Crunch up and to the left until your right elbow touches your left knee, then slowly return to the start position. Repeat for reps, then switch sides.

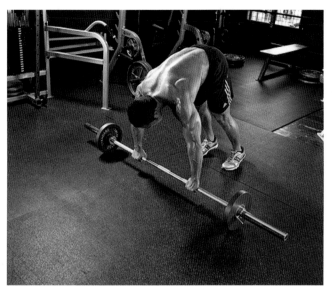

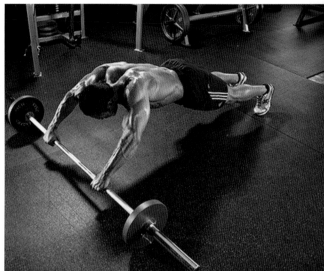

AB ROLLOUT

START: Place a barbell with circular plates on the floor so it can roll back and forth. Use a shoulder-width grip and begin either bent over with your legs extended and the bar in front of your shins or kneeling with the bar right in front of you. (The standing position is extremely advanced; most people will need to start in the kneeling position.)

EXECUTION: Slowly roll the bar forward until your torso is nearly parallel to the floor, then contract your abs to roll the bar back toward you. Don't let your hips sag.

MONDAY | LEGS, ABS
A.M.
"High" Cardio

This workout comprises a six-move dumbbell circuit and four treadmill intervals superset with explosive exercises. Choose relatively light weights. *For the complete workout, see page 31.*

P.M.

EXERCISE	WEEKS 1-3 SETS	REPS	WEEKS 4-6 SETS	REPS
LEGS				
Barbell Squat (warmup)	2[1]	10	2[1]	10
Barbell Squat (continued)	3[2] 5[3]	5 10	5[4]	5
Romanian Deadlift	2	20	2	20
Lying or Seated Leg Curl	3	15	3	15
ABS				
Platehead Decline Situp	5	10	5	12

Rest 90 seconds between sets of squats and 45–60 seconds between sets of all other exercises.
1 RESISTANCE — Set 1: 30% of one-rep max (1RM); Set 2: 40% 1RM
2 RESISTANCE — Set 1: 60% 1RM; Set 2: 70% 1RM; Set 3: 80% 1RM
3 RESISTANCE — all sets: 30%–40% 1RM (go light enough that you can do 10 reps per set)
4 RESISTANCE — all sets: 60% 1RM

TUESDAY | CHEST, BACK, ABS
A.M.

EXERCISE	WEEKS 1-3 SETS	REPS	WEEKS 4-6 SETS	REPS
CHEST				
Barbell Bench Press (warmup)	2[1]	10	2[1]	10
Barbell Bench Press (contd.)	3[2] 5[3]	5 10	5[6]	5
BACK				
Inverted Row		50[4]		50[4]
Barbell Bentover Row	3	12	3	15
J-pull	3	12	3	15
ABS				
20/20 Ab Circuit[5]:				
Feet-elevated Crunch		20		20
Figure-4 Crunch		10/side		10/side
Skywalker		20		20

Rest 90 seconds between sets of bench presses and 45–60 seconds between sets of all other exercises.
1 RESISTANCE — Set 1: 30% 1RM; Set 2: 40% 1RM
2 RESISTANCE — Set 1: 60% 1RM; Set 2: 70% 1RM; Set 3: 80% 1RM
3 RESISTANCE — all sets: 30%-40% (go light enough that you can do 10 reps per set)
4 Do 50 total reps in the fewest number of sets possible.
5 Do 20 reps on, 20 seconds off, alternating between the feet-elevated crunch, figure-4 crunch, and skywalker for as many rounds as possible.
6 RESISTANCE — all sets: 60% 1RM

P.M.
"Moderate" Cardio

This routine includes an upper-body resistance-band circuit and a weighted plyometric exercise. *For the complete workout, see page 32.*

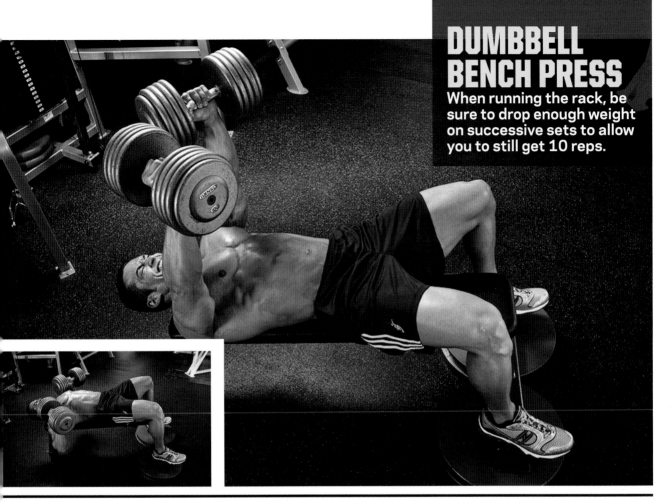

When running the rack, be sure to drop enough weight on successive sets to allow you to still get 10 reps.

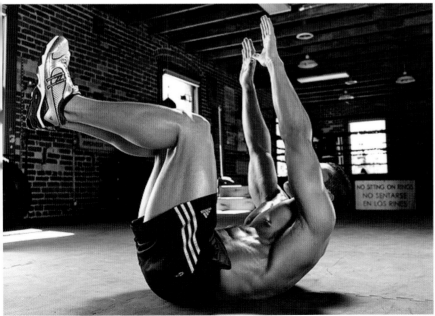

FEET-ELEVATED CRUNCH

START: Lie faceup on the floor with your feet in the air, and your hips and knees bent 90 degrees. Extend your arms toward the ceiling.

EXECUTION: Keeping your hips and knees bent and your feet up, contract your abs to lift your shoulder blades off the floor and raise your hands toward the ceiling. Squeeze your abs hard, then lower back to the floor.

SPLITTING FIBERS

NO ONE SAID getting a six-pack was going to be easy. The lifting will be intense, as will the cardio (see "Burning Down the House" on page 30), but to get the full benefits of each it's best to divide them into separate training sessions with at least four to six hours and a few meals in between. It's the classic a.m./p.m. split, with one workout taking place before work or school and the other later in the evening.

Lifting and cardio alternate between a.m. and p.m. sessions. Low-intensity, steady-state cardio is always done first thing in the morning on an empty stomach, which has been proven to burn more fat than when it's done at other times of the day. High-intensity interval training (HIIT) is also positioned in the morning, since doing it after a hard leg workout would diminish the gains made with squats and other lower-body moves. Moderate-intensity cardio will be done in the afternoon on days when you lift in the morning.

If six weeks of two-a-days isn't feasible in your schedule, feel free to do weights and cardio in the same session, even though that's not ideal. Here's why: Since the primary goal of this program is getting lean, the focus shifts somewhat to the HIIT workouts, and you don't want your lifting to be counterproductive. Consider the glycogen stores the body uses during each training session: If you lift weights and then have a post-workout meal, you're in an anabolic state. If you lift weights and then use an entirely different energy system to do cardio, you essentially zap all the glycogen stores you need after lifting, rendering you much less anabolic. The more anabolic you are, the faster your metabolism and vice versa.

It's no accident that your hardest lifting workout (legs) and toughest cardio session (HIIT) fall on the same days: Monday and Thursday. Your body needs time to recover from the most taxing workouts,

and doing legs and HIIT on consecutive days won't allow for this. The other training days in the split, when all lifting is upper-body and cardio is moderate and low-intensity, will act as an active rest following your grueling lower-body/HIIT days.

Lifting and cardio will consume the vast majority of your time and attention in the gym, but direct ab work shouldn't be an afterthought. Train abs as part of every weight-room workout six days a week.

Our six moves will hit your abs from multiple angles with varying rep schemes and resistance to promote hypertrophy, endurance and core stability, thus providing both aesthetic and functional benefits.

The lifting program as a whole, combined with proper nutrition and cardio, is guaranteed to reveal a better, stronger, and more visible six-pack. See if your plastic infomercial gadget can do that.

WEDNESDAY | TRICEPS, BICEPS, DELTS, ABS

A.M.
"Low" Cardio
Set a treadmill to an 8%–10% incline and walk at a moderate pace for 20-30 minutes. *For the complete workout, see page 30.*

P.M.

	WEEKS 1–3		WEEKS 4–6	
EXERCISE	**SETS**	**REPS/TIME**	**SETS**	**REPS/TIME**
TRICEPS				
Bench Dip		50[1]		50[1]
Rope Pushdown	3	12	3	15
Rope Overhead				
Triceps Extension	3	12	3	15
BICEPS				
Barbell Curl	3	12	3	12
Hammer Curl				
(run the rack)		10		10
+ Static Plate				
Hold[2]	1	30 sec.	1	30 sec.
DELTS				
Leaning Dumbbell				
Lateral Raise	3	12	3	12
ABS				
Ab Rollout	3	10	3	10
—superset with—				
Plank	3	30 sec.	3	30 sec.

Rest 30 seconds between all sets.
1 Do 50 total reps in the fewest number of sets possible.
2 On hammer curls, do dropsets of 10 reps each, starting with the heaviest dumbbells you can use for 10 reps and dropping the weight each set until you can no longer do 10 reps. Immediately hold a weight plate with both hands in the middle of a curl (elbows bent 90 degrees, forearms parallel to the floor) for 30 seconds.

J-PULL
Pull a rope or V-bar from the high-pulley cable toward your a[...] in a J-shaped path. Squeeze your shoul[...]der blades together at the bottom of each rep.

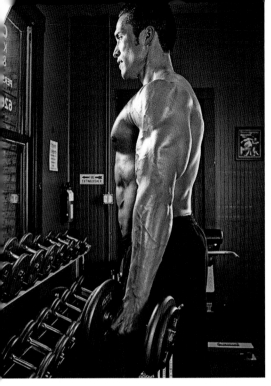
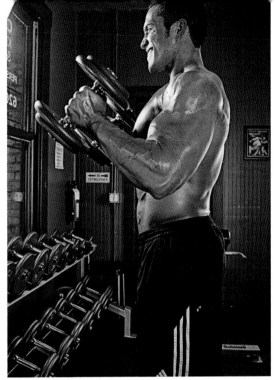

HAMMER CURL (RUN THE RACK) + STATIC PLATE HOLD

After as many drop-sets of 10 hammer curls as you can do, hold a weight plate in a half-way-up curl position for 30 seconds.

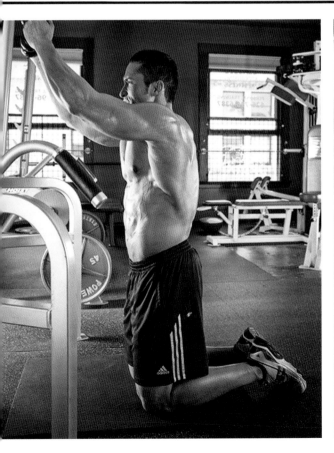
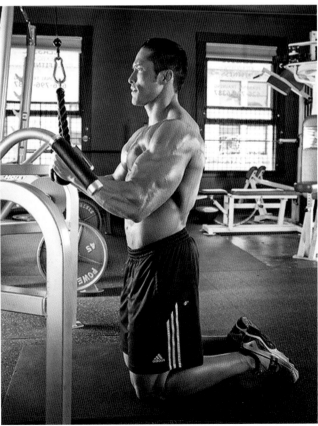

THURSDAY I POSTERIOR CHAIN, ABS
A.M.
"High" Cardio
For the complete workout, see page 31.

P.M.

EXERCISE	WEEKS 1-3 SETS	REPS	WEEKS 4-6 SETS	REPS
POSTERIOR CHAIN				
Barbell Deadlift				
(warmup)	2[1]	10	2[1]	10
Barbell Deadlift	3[2]	5	5[3]	5
Romanian				
Deadlift	5	10	2	20
Barbell Shrug	3	15	3	15
Lying or Seated				
Leg Curl	3	15	3	15
ABS				
Platehead				
Decline Situp	5	10	5	10

Rest 90 seconds between sets of deadlifts and 45-60 seconds between sets of all other exercises.
1 RESISTANCE — Set 1: 30% 1RM; Set 2: 40% 1RM
2 RESISTANCE — Set 1: 60% 1RM; Set 2: 70% 1RM; Set 3: 80% 1RM
3 RESISTANCE — all sets: 60% 1RM

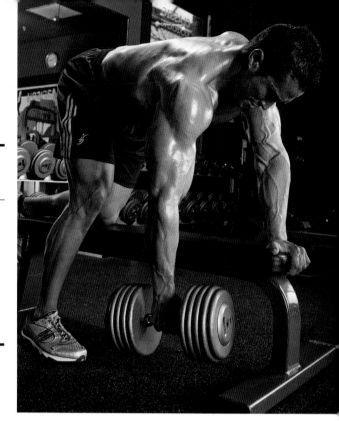

FRIDAY I CHEST, BACK, ABS
A.M.

EXERCISE	WEEKS 1-3 SETS	REPS	WEEKS 4-6 SETS	REPS
CHEST				
Dumbbell				
Bench Press				
(run the rack)[1]		10		10
Cable Crossover	3	15	3	15
BACK				
Kroc Row[2]	1	To failure	1	To failure
Chest-Supported				
Row	3	12	3	12
J-pull	3	12	3	12
ABS				
20/20 Ab Circuit:[3]				
Feet-elevated				
Crunch		20		20
Figure-4 Crunch		10/side		10/side
Skywalker		20		20

Rest 45-60 seconds between all sets.
1 Do dropsets of 10 reps each, starting with the heaviest dumbbells you can use for 10 reps and dropping the weight each set until you can no longer do 10 reps.
2 Select a dumbbell with which you think you can do 15-20 reps and do as many reps of one-arm rows as possible with each arm. The next week, try to surpass that number.
3 Do 20 reps on, 20 seconds off, alternating between feet-elevated crunches, figure-4 crunches and skywalkers for as many rounds as possible.

P.M.
"Moderate" Cardio
For the complete workout, see page 32.

SATURDAY I TRICEPS, BICEPS, DELTS, ABS
A.M.
"Low" Cardio
For the complete workout, see page 32.

P.M.

EXERCISE	WEEKS 1-3 SETS	REPS/TIME	WEEKS 4-6 SETS	REPS/TIME
TRICEPS				
Bench Dip		50[1]		50[1]
Rope Pushdown	3	12	3	15
Rope Overhead				
Triceps Extension	3	12	3	15
BICEPS				
Barbell Curl	3	12	3	12
Hammer Curl[2]				
(run the rack)		10		10
+ Static Plate				
Hold[2]	1	30 sec.	1	30 sec.
DELTS				
Leaning Dumbbell				
Lateral Raise	3	12	3	12
ABS				
Ab Rollout	3	10	3	10
—superset with—				
Plank	3	30 sec.	3	30 sec.

Rest 30 seconds between all sets.
1 Do 50 total reps in the fewest number of sets possible.
2 On hammer curls, do dropsets of 10 reps each, starting with the heaviest dumbbells you can use for 10 reps and dropping the weight each set until you can no longer do 10 reps. Immediately hold a weight plate with both hands in the middle of a curl (elbows bent 90 degrees, forearms parallel to the floor) for 30 seconds.

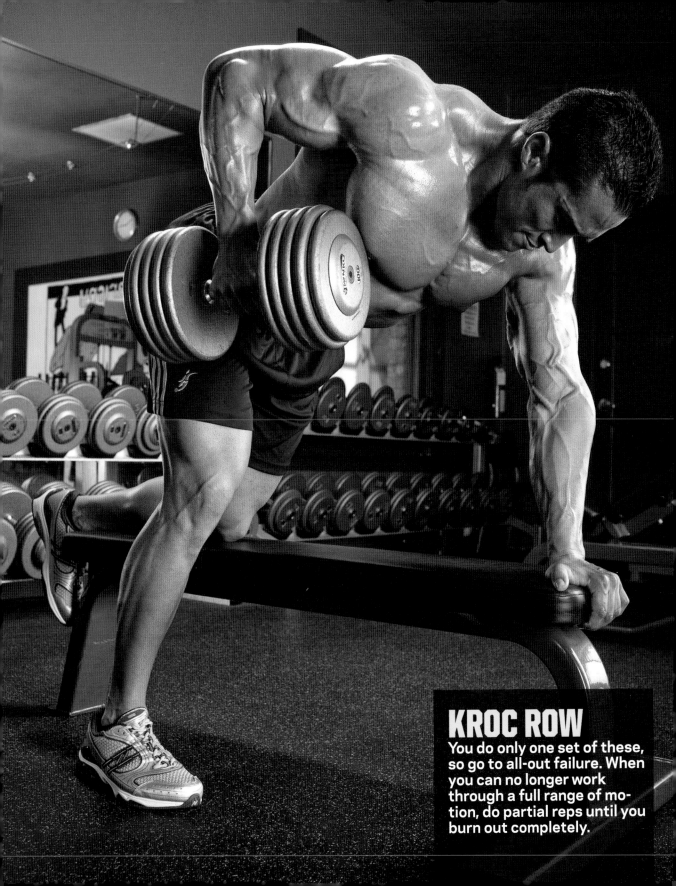

KROC ROW
You do only one set of these, so go to all-out failure. When you can no longer work through a full range of motion, do partial reps until you burn out completely.

BURNING DOWN

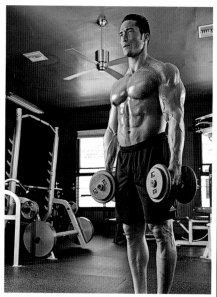

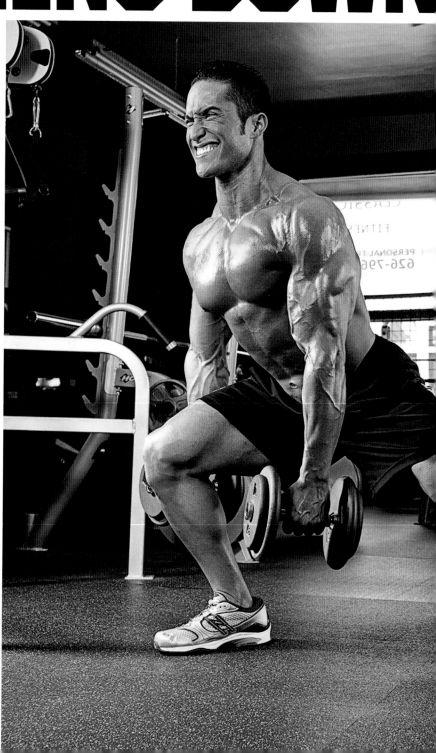

SHED FAT LIKE A FIGHTER WITH THIS RADICAL THREE-PRONGED CARDIO ROUTINE

For the fastest possible fat-burning results, you need a cardio plan that breaks a few rules. We've enlisted Kelly Tekin, M.S., C.S.C.S.—a competitive bodybuilder and strength and conditioning coach whose client list includes UFC fighters Rashad Evans, Jon "Bones" Jones, and James McSweeney—to design three MMA-inspired routines that'll push conventional boundaries and strip fat from your midsection. Tekin's high-, moderate-, and low-intensity routines challenge your aerobic capacity with circuits containing a variety of athletically functional movements. "Each circuit is designed to be performed at the pace fighters use to prepare for a match," she says of the program's ferocious training tempo. "By forcing your body to work explosively with little rest, you'll not only burn body fat faster but also train all your muscle fibers to fire faster."

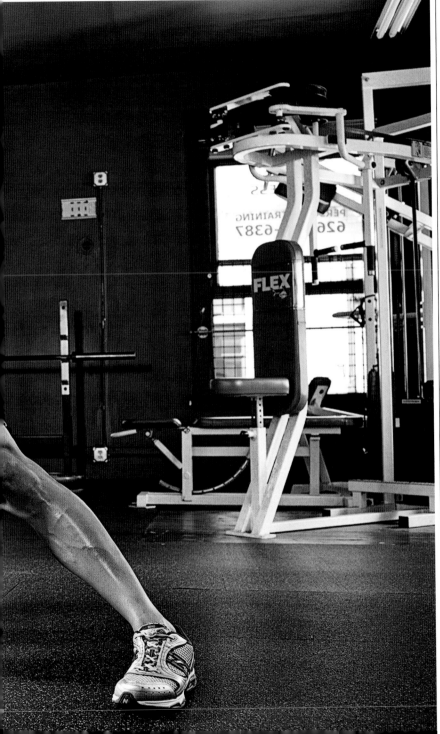

HE HOUSE

HIGH-INTENSITY DAY
MONDAY, THURSDAY

The most difficult workout of this series comprises a six-move dumbbell circuit and four treadmill intervals superset with explosive exercises. Tekin suggests choosing relatively light weights for the dumbbell circuit to provide just enough resistance to make it challenging.

For the treadmill intervals, you'll jog for 30 seconds and sprint for 30 seconds, repeating for a total of four minutes. After each interval, you'll perform the prescribed exercise, then immediately jump back on the treadmill for the next interval.

PART 1

EXERCISE	REPS
Dumbbell Reverse Lunge	6 each leg
Dumbbell Stiff-leg Deadlift	12
Dumbbell Jump Squat	12
Dumbbell Front Squat	6
Dumbbell Lateral Lunge	6 each leg
Dumbbell Push-press	6

Rest 40–60 seconds after each round. Complete six circuits.

PART 2

EXERCISE	REPS/TIME
Treadmill Interval	4 min.
Medicine Ball Slam	20
Treadmill Interval	4 min.
Power Pullup	20
Treadmill Interval	4 min.
Split-Squat Jump	10 each leg
Treadmill Interval	4 min.
One-arm Dumbbell Swing	10 each arm

Perform exercises in order with no rest in between.

DUMBBELL LATERAL LUNGE

Stand erect with a dumbbell in each hand. Take a large step to one side and bend your knee to lower your body. Keep your trailing leg fully extended. Return to the start by powerfully extending your lead knee and hip. Repeat on the other side.

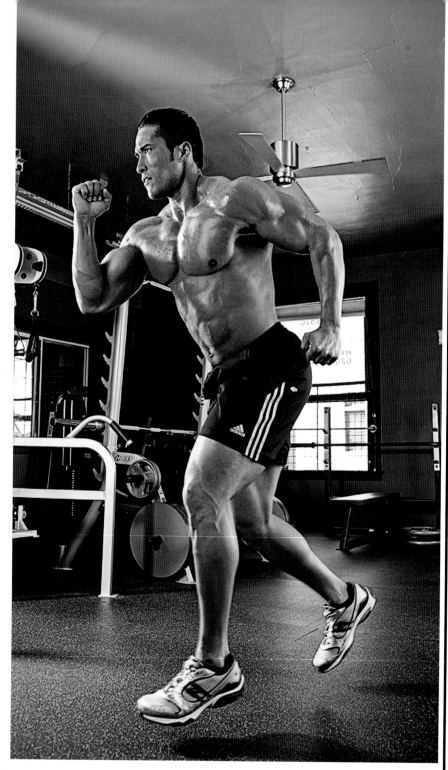

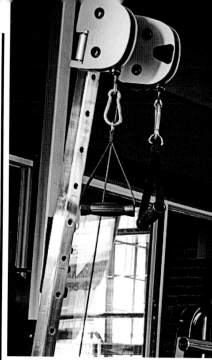

MODERATE-INTENSITY DAY
TUESDAY, FRIDAY

This workout includes an upper-body resistance-band circuit and a weighted plyometric exercise. For the circuit, attach one end of two resistance bands to the base of a sturdy object, such as a bench or power rack.

After completing all rounds of the circuit, rest two minutes before doing the weighted-vest jumps. "If you don't have a weighted vest, spend double the time jumping (60 seconds) during each set. Keep the rest periods to two minutes," Tekin says.

EXERCISE	REPS
Power Band	30
Alternating Band Row	30
Band Oblique Twist	30 each side
Band Punch	30 each arm
Band Upright Row + Jump	30

Rest 60 seconds after each round. Complete five circuits.

Weighted-Vest Jump
Do 3 sets of 30 seconds, resting two minutes in between.

LOW-INTENSITY DAY
WEDNESDAY, SATURDAY

Set a treadmill to an 8%–10% incline and walk at a moderate pace for 20–30 minutes. "This will give your muscles time to recover from the other workouts as well as burn more body fat," Tekin explains.

SPLIT-SQUAT JUMP

Get into a one-leg squat position: one leg forward, knee bent 90 degrees, and thigh parallel to the floor. Explosively extend your working knee and hip, and jump, switching legs midair. Land in a one-leg squat with your other leg forward.

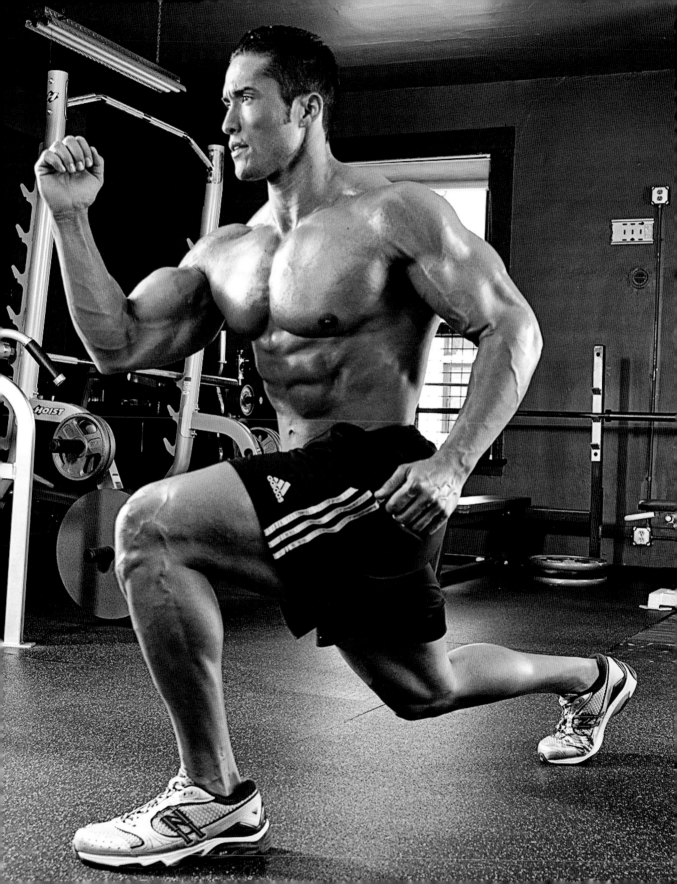

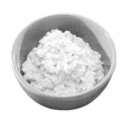
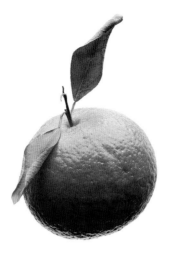
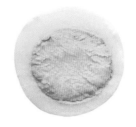
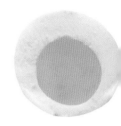

FEED YOUR ABS

IF YOU WANT A SIX-PACK IN SIX WEEKS, YOU HAVE TO **EAT RIGHT.** HERE'S HOW TO DO IT.

Your road to washboard abs is divided into two nutritional phases. Phase 1 (Weeks 1-3) is designed to shift your body into fat-burning mode by establishing a solid foundation. Phase 2 (Weeks 4-6) builds on the principles presented in Phase 1 but further reduces calorie and carb levels to push your body to accelerate fat loss. Follow the advice presented here and you'll be well on your way to a chiseled core.

1/ GO MICRO
> Getting lean takes more than just modifying your protein, carb, and fat intake. You also need to pay attention to the little things. For example:

STAY HYDRATED Believe it or not, drinking water plays a huge role in your efforts to burn fat and maintain lean mass. Good hydration speeds the metabolism, helps reduce hunger, flushes the body of toxins, and aids in muscle growth and repair. Keeping yourself properly hydrated should be top priority when you're trying to reveal your abs. Aim to consume about one gallon of water per day.

MILK THE BURN High-calcium diets from low-fat dairy products have been shown to boost fat loss, specifically around the abs. Researchers from the University of Tennessee-Knoxville found that subjects on such a diet lost more total body fat and abdominal fat than those on a low-calcium diet. Reach for Greek or other varieties of yogurt, low-fat cheese, cottage cheese, and milk to boost your calcium and protein intake.

C RESULTS Ramp up your vitamin C intake and watch the fat slide right off. Research shows that individuals with adequate vitamin C status (500 milligrams a day) burn 25% more body fat during exercise than those with low levels of C. Choose vitamin C-rich foods such as apples, bell peppers, berries, broccoli, citrus fruits, leafy greens, and tomatoes.

2/ SLASH CALORIES
> The first step on the road to a great midsection is to establish an appropriate calorie level to initiate fat loss. To do so, you must create a caloric deficit by burning more calories than you consume. Once this deficit is achieved the body will tap into fat reserves to provide the energy needed to fuel your workouts and daily activity.

>> **PHASE 1:** Consume 15 calories per pound of body weight. For a 180-pounder, that's 2,700 calories per day. To keep your metabolism burning at full flame, eat a meal every 2–3 hours for a total of at least six meals per day.

>> **PHASE 2:** Cut your intake to 13 calories per pound, which comes to 2,340 calories per day for a 180-pound guy. This creates a greater caloric deficit and further enhances your fat-loss potential.

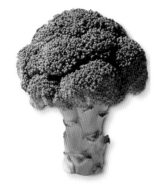
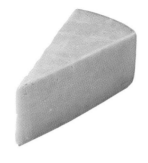
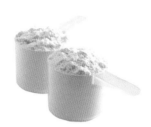
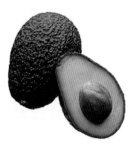

3/ PUSH PROTEIN

> The war against fat includes more than just mercilessly cutting calories. For starters, not all calories are created equal. The body burns twice as many calories while digesting protein compared to carbs and almost 30% more than fat. Besides boosting metabolism and blunting hunger, high-protein diets also help preserve lean muscle. This becomes an important factor when you reduce calories and carbs so the body doesn't burn muscle for energy. Choose high-quality sources such as eggs and egg whites, fish, lean steak, low-fat dairy, pork tenderloin, and skinless chicken and turkey breast, as well as casein, soy, and whey protein powders.

>> PHASE 1: Ignite your body's metabolic fire by consuming 1–1.5 grams of protein per pound of bodyweight (180–270 grams a day for our 180-pounder). Keep your intake consistent during the day, ingesting about 30 grams at each meal.

>> PHASE 2: During this reduction phase, protein intake must remain high to help preserve muscle. Increase your levels to 1.5–2 grams per pound (270–360 grams per day for the 180-pound trainee).

4/ EAT HEALTHY FATS

> For years this nutrient has been considered a dietary demon, but healthy fats can be very beneficial in shedding that top layer of blubber. Several studies indicate that healthy fats from monounsaturated and omega-3 sources not only promote fat loss but also increase satiety, so you feel full longer. As a bonus, healthy fats aid in the recovery process, fighting off inflammation induced by hard training.

>> PHASES 1 AND 2: Dietary fat should make up 20%–30% of your total daily calories. Amounts will vary depending on your carb intake for the day. On low-carb days, fat intake increases to 30% of your total calories; on high-carb days, levels drop to about 20%. Emphasize monounsaturated sources such as almonds, avocados, olive oil, and peanut butter, and omega-3 fats such as flaxseeds, salmon, and walnuts.

5/ CYCLE CARBS

> Manipulating your carb intake not only helps you cut calories but also allows you to exert some hormonal control. The key to being able to melt away fat and inhibit the storage of body fat is keeping insulin levels in check. Eating fast-digesting carbs (such as sports drinks, white bread, and white potatoes) spikes insulin levels and halts fat burning while accelerating fat storage. On the flip side, slow-digesting carbs cause a less dramatic rise in insulin and provide long-lasting energy. The only time fast carbs reign supreme is immediately post-workout, when the insulin spike helps replenish glycogen stores and kick-starts muscle-protein synthesis. Other than post-workout, always select slow carbs such as brown rice, legumes, oatmeal, sweet potatoes, whole grains, and whole fruits and vegetables.

Take your body to the next level of lean by alternating high- and low-carb days. Known as carb cycling, this prevents the body from adapting to one consistent level of intake. As a result of this cycling, your metabolic rate remains high and fat is continuously thrown on the furnace. Furthermore, high-carb days will help recharge energy levels and aid in the recovery process from high-intensity workouts.

>> PHASE 1: Carb intake ranges from 1–1.5 grams per pound of body weight, totaling 180–270 grams per day for the 180-pounder. On high-intensity workout days (Days 1, 4, and 6), increase your carbs to the higher end of the spectrum; on lower-intensity workout days (Days 2, 3, 5, and 7), drop your carbs to the lower end of the range.

>> PHASE 2: Continue with the same cyclic approach using a carb spectrum that shrinks to 0.5–1 gram per pound of body weight. This creates a greater caloric deficit and continues to force the body to utilize fat stores for energy. On low-carb days, the 180-pound guy would limit his intake to about 90 grams while striving for the higher end of the recommended protein range. On high-carb days, levels may increase up to 180 grams.

CHAPTER 3

THE
METABOLIC
WORKOUT

STRIP OFF EXCESS BODY FAT AND TAKE YOUR CONDITIONING TO THE NEXT LEVEL WITH METABOLIC CIRCUIT TRAINING

The excess fat on your body is a lot like a nut attached to a rusted-out bolt. You want to twist it off. You need to twist it off. Chances are, you've tried everything you can think of to unscrew it, but nothing ever seems to work. It's stuck—and so are you.

When this happens, any machine or auto repair shop worth its salt has just the last-resort solution on hand to get things moving: a blowtorch. When you blowtorch a rusted nut-and-bolt arrangement, the intense heat breaks the bond created by the rust, and it melts things down to a point where the nut can easily be removed.

That's how it works with fat loss, too. When all else fails—when your current diet and cardio practices aren't solving a blessed thing—it's time to break out your own blowtorch and get the lard off once and for all. We're about to show you how to burn off that last bit of stubborn body fat with a healthy dose of intensity by adding metabolic circuit training to your regimen.

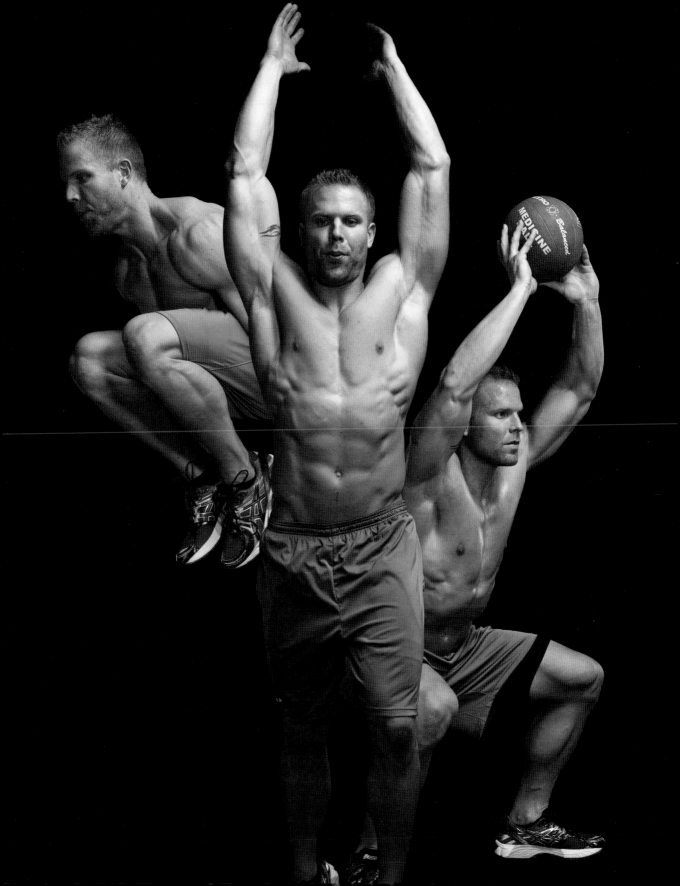

EPOC EPIC

You may have heard about excess post-exercise oxygen consumption in the past. EPOC is the gas tank that powers your fat-stripping blowtorch, because when the type of training we're advocating here induces an "oxygen debt," it can increase your metabolic rate for up to 16 hours after you train. This means that when you're done working out—while you're at school, at work, or sleeping—your body is still looking to consume fuel sources for the oxygen it needs to restore itself to a resting state of equilibrium. The good news for you is that it does this primarily through raiding fat stores.

"The EPOC effect does what steady-state cardio can't do," says Ryan Whitton, a strength coach in Austin, TX. "You still need some steady-state in your program to enhance recovery and strengthen your heart, but when it comes to stripping fat off your body, nothing works like circuit training to manipulate the speed at which your metabolism burns."

Research shows that the EPOC effect increases along with the intensity level of the type of exercise you're performing. So, while you may burn more calories during a low-impact 45-minute treadmill session, you'll affect your metabolic rate in a far more profound way if you throw in two or three short-yet-intense 10-minute metabolic circuits per week.

SHREDDED FOR SUMMER

Whether you're willing to admit it or not, metabolic-style training is fun despite its high degree of difficulty. The workouts move quickly, the exercises are constantly changing, and it forces you to use your entire body as a unit—the way it's intended to move—instead of performing the same repetitive moves for set periods of time, à la steady-state cardio.

You can also train this way anywhere. Whether you're traveling or pressed for time, or you'd rather wait until you're home from the gym to receive your metabolic ass kicking, most of the exercises in this set of workouts involve just your body weight—with the rest utilizing dumbbells, the weight of which can remain constant. In other words, you won't need a ton of time, space, or gear—just the desire to shred those last bits of winter body fat and a plan to complete the job.

"If I showed you someone who trained with these circuits for an extended period of time," says Whitton, an experienced amateur fighter who favors MMA-style training for his clients, "you'd see how they look and perform and you'd want those types of results for yourself. If you want to be lean for summer, and you want the kinesthetic awareness to control your own body, this is how it's done."

HOW IT WORKS

Perform circuits consecutively with no breaks between exercises; then rest for 60 to 90 seconds between rounds—crank out as many rounds as you can.

This doesn't mean you should be hitting these circuits every day, however. For most people, two or three hard metabolic circuits per week will suffice, because you can't recover from this level of intensity in just 24 hours. Additionally, the hampered recovery levels caused by overtraining with metabolic circuits will negatively affect your strength and mass-building workouts, because you won't be recovered enough to make significant progress if you're consistently running yourself into the ground with anaerobic torture. Your body can't hold up to it, and your returns will begin to diminish in short order.

"The best way to get this done is to leave at least 48 to 72 hours between workouts," Whitton says. "Too many guys think that if they're not in a constant state of exhaustion they're not going to burn enough fat, but this isn't the case. These workouts are about quality as much as quantity. I'd rather see my clients work themselves to exhaustion twice per week and take the rest of the days off than train like this every day, because all the positive changes to your body happen during recovery periods."

Now, this won't be an easy six weeks. You'll essentially be working yourself to the bone twice per week—getting more rounds in each time out—in order to accelerate your results, so this isn't a "less is more" training scenario. That's a good thing, according to Whitton. "Along with basking in the glow of the EPOC effect," he says, "when you eventually get off the floor and leave the gym, you know you put in a hard day's work, and that's worth all the effort."

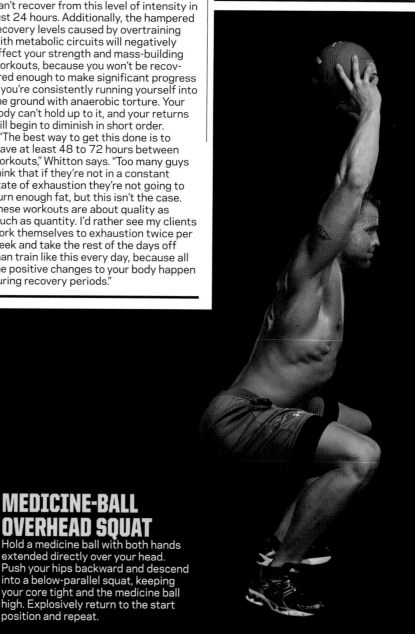

MEDICINE-BALL OVERHEAD SQUAT

Hold a medicine ball with both hands extended directly over your head. Push your hips backward and descend into a below-parallel squat, keeping your core tight and the medicine ball high. Explosively return to the start position and repeat.

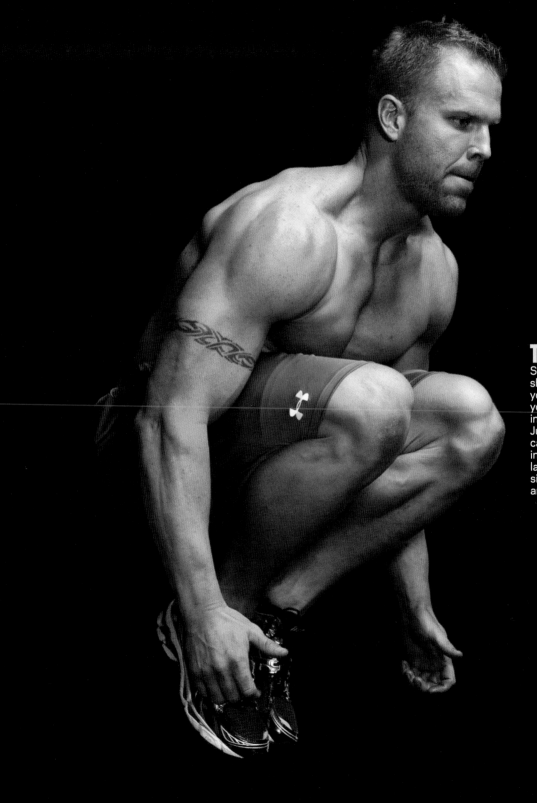

TUCK JUMP

Stand with your feet shoulder-width apart, your knees bent, and your hands and elbows in an athletic position. Jump as high as you can, tuck your knees into your chest, then land as softly as possible. Gather yourself and repeat for reps.

BURPEE WITH TUCK JUMP

From a standing position, squat down, place your hands on the floor and kick your feet back simultaneously so you're in a pushup position. Rapidly bring your feet back to the squat position, then explode upward into a tuck jump, bringing your knees up to your chest. Repeat.

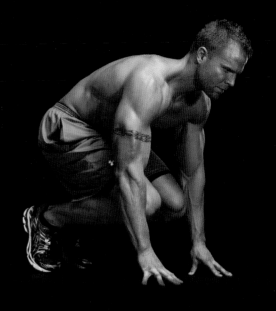

FIGURE-4 SITUP

Lie on the floor on your back, with your knees bent. Cross one leg over the other so the outside of your elevated leg, just above your ankle, is resting on your other leg just above the knee. Place your hand opposite your elevated leg behind your head, then bend at the waist and try to touch your elbow to your elevated knee. Repeat for reps on both sides.

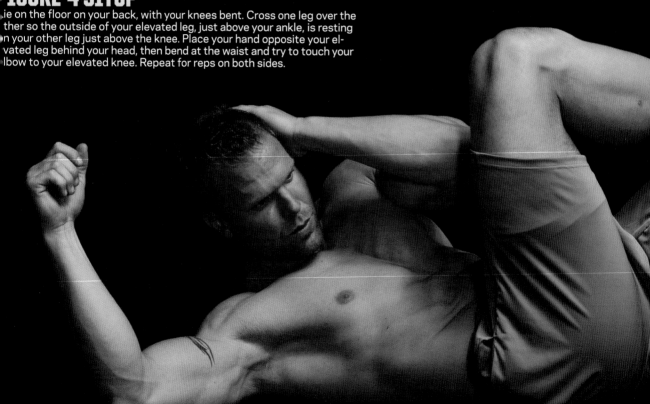

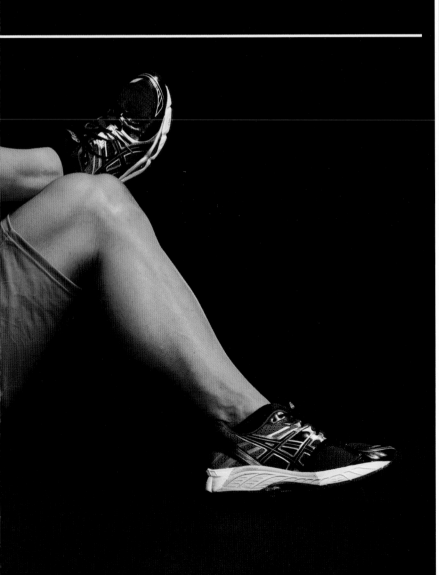

Two or three times per week, choose one of the following workouts and perform as many rounds as you can.

EXERCISE	REPS
Medicine Ball Overhead Squat	10
Tuck Jump	10
Scissor Lunge	10
Skip and Scoop	20 yards there and back
Burpee with Tuck Jump	10
Pushup	10
Mountain Climber	10
Figure-4 Situp	10 each side
DB Burpee Clean and Press	10
DB Thruster	10
DB Snatch	10 each hand
DB Woodchopper	10 each side

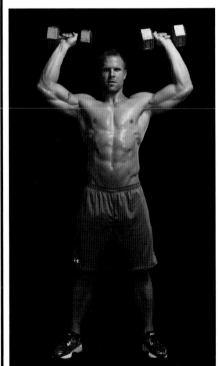

DUMBBELL BURPEE CLEAN AND PRESS

Holding a pair of dumbbells, perform a burpee except without the tuck jump. Once you've returned to the start position, explosively clean the dumbbells to shoulder level, then press them over your head. Lower the weights to your sides and repeat.

MOUNTAIN CLIMBER

Stay in a pushup position and forcefully kick your left knee to your chest, landing the ball of your left foot on the ground. Then, bring your right knee to your chest and return your right foot to the start position. Repeat as though you were running in place.

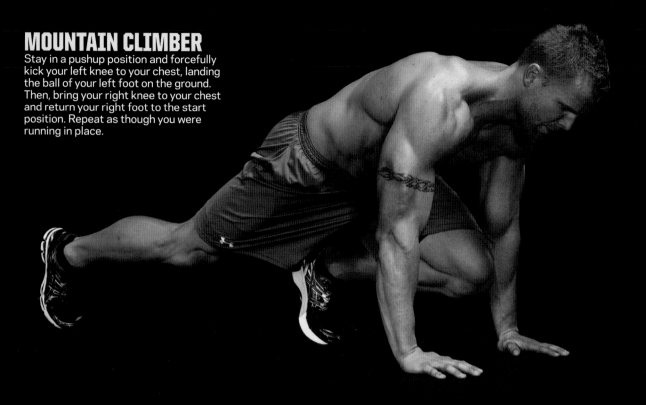

DUMBBELL SNATCH

Stand with your feet shoulder-width apart and your knees slightly bent, holding a dumbbell in front of each thigh. Extend your ankles, knees, and hips to explosively raise both dumbbells overhead. You should feel like you're trying to throw them through the ceiling.

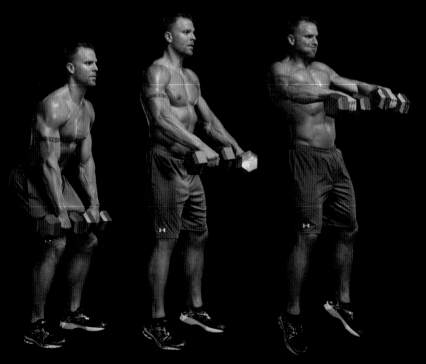

SKIP AND SCOOP

From a standing position, move forward by driving your right knee into your chest to begin the skip. Land on the ball of your left foot, then immediately descend into a lunge with your right foot forward. From this position, explode into another skip, this time leading with your left knee. Repeat for 20 yards down and back.

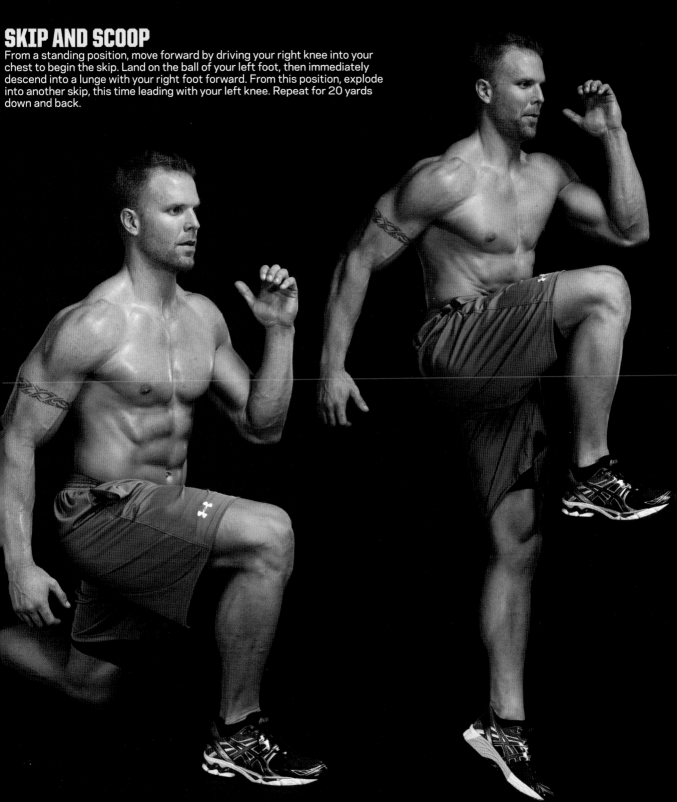

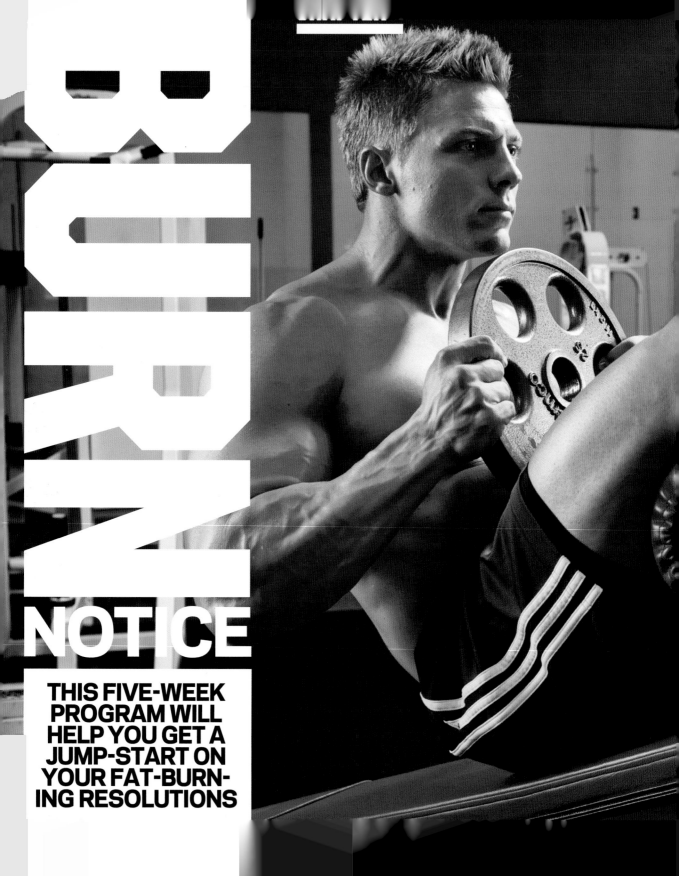

BURN
NOTICE

THIS FIVE-WEEK PROGRAM WILL HELP YOU GET A JUMP-START ON YOUR FAT-BURNING RESOLUTIONS

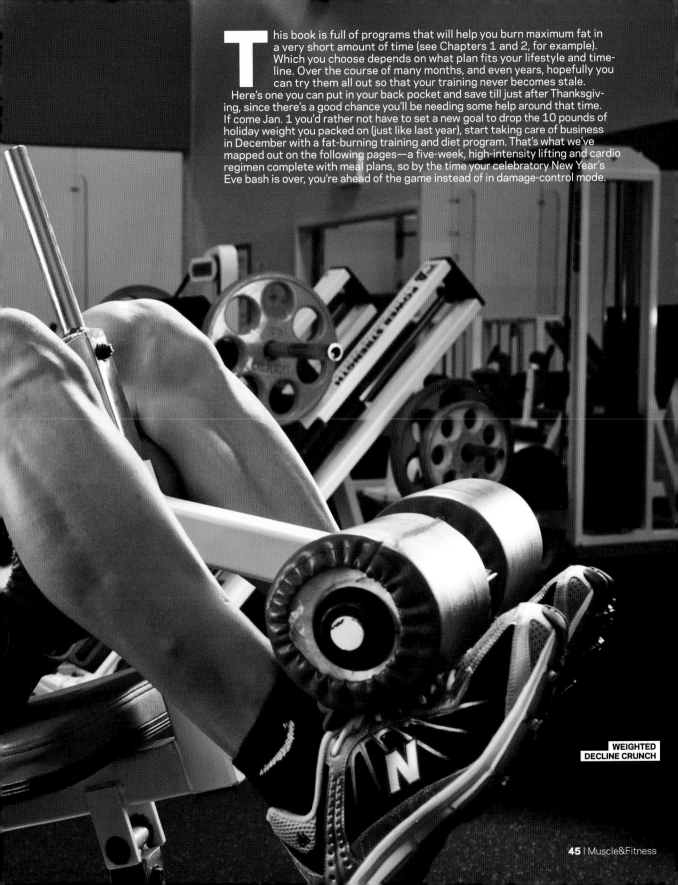

This book is full of programs that will help you burn maximum fat in a very short amount of time (see Chapters 1 and 2, for example). Which you choose depends on what plan fits your lifestyle and time-line. Over the course of many months, and even years, hopefully you can try them all out so that your training never becomes stale.

Here's one you can put in your back pocket and save till just after Thanksgiving, since there's a good chance you'll be needing some help around that time. If come Jan. 1 you'd rather not have to set a new goal to drop the 10 pounds of holiday weight you packed on (just like last year), start taking care of business in December with a fat-burning training and diet program. That's what we've mapped out on the following pages—a five-week, high-intensity lifting and cardio regimen complete with meal plans, so by the time your celebratory New Year's Eve bash is over, you're ahead of the game instead of in damage-control mode.

WEIGHTED DECLINE CRUNCH

SHREDDING SEASON

IF YOU'RE GOING through the motions in your current workouts, you'll immediately notice one change when you under-take this program: Intensity is going to increase. Not necessarily in terms of heavier weights but rather in the application of advanced training techniques such as dropsets, forced reps, and partial reps that'll take your muscles past the point of failure, and supersets that'll speed up your training pace to increase calorie-burning. The degree of change you'll see will be directly proportional to the amount of intensity you apply toward the program; in other words, if you slack off, your ultimate potential will be limited. Consistency is your key to success. Given the shortened timetable, it's imperative you don't skip any workouts.

In this program you'll weight-train three days a week in the first three weeks, then increase that frequency to four days a week in the final two weeks, in addition to cardio workouts (see "Cardio Component" sidebar). Sets and reps are based on a light-to-heavy pyramid system. On compound exercises such as presses and squats, your first set employs higher reps with lighter weight; and successive sets will be heavier, so choose a weight that allows you to reach muscular failure at the rep indicated. Later in the workouts, when mostly isolation exercises are being used, rep counts won't pyramid and weight can stay the same.

To keep the intensity level high during the routine, be strict with your rest periods. In the first three weeks, rest no longer than one minute between sets. (Within supersets—of which there will be plenty—you won't rest at all.) In Weeks 4 and 5, reduce rest to 45 seconds. If you rest too long, your heart rate slows and fat-burning potential is diminished, so maintain a quick pace throughout. The short rest periods and advanced training techniques will maximize your metabolism, which is what makes a leaner, more shredded physique possible.

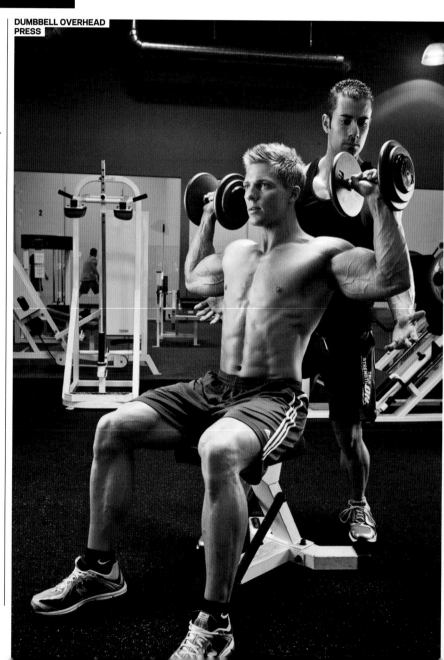

DUMBBELL OVERHEAD PRESS

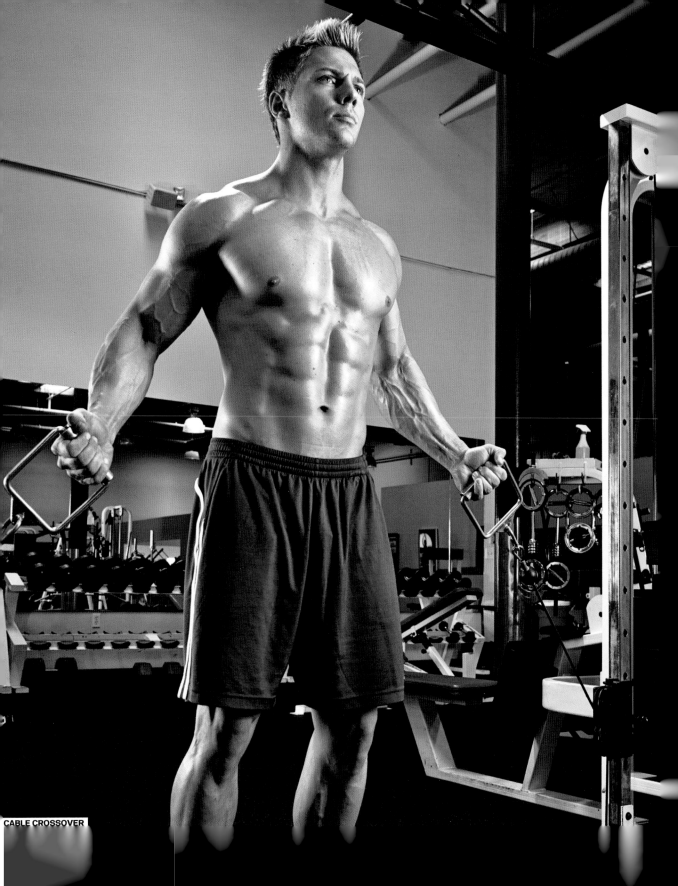

CABLE CROSSOVER

5-WEEK FAT-BURNING

START with a 5-10-minute warmup on the cardio equipment of your choice.

DURING Weeks 1–3, rest 60 seconds between sets. In Weeks 4 and 5, cut your rest periods to 45 seconds while still striving to lift the same amount of weight for the same number of reps.

EXTEND your set where indicated with advanced training principles. These include:

SUPERSETS
Perform exercises back to back with no rest.

FORCED REPS
A training partner provides assistance, allowing you to complete a few extra reps past failure.

DROPSETS
Once you reach muscle failure, quickly drop the weight by 20%-30% and continue doing as many reps as you can until you reach failure again. At that point, reduce the weight again and go to failure once more.

PARTIAL REPS
After you reach muscle failure, complete several additional reps by powering through a very short range of motion.

PRE-EXHAUST
Complete a single-joint exercise before a compound movement to pre-fatigue the target muscle group.

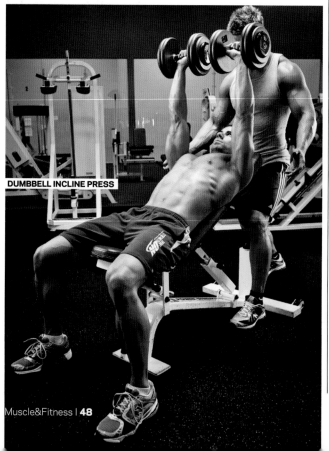

DUMBBELL INCLINE PRESS

THE WORKOUT—WEEKS 1-3

MONDAY: CHEST, BACK, ABS

EXERCISE	SETS	REPS	ADVANCED TECHNIQUE
BENCH PRESS	4	12,10,8,8	Supersets
—superset with—			
BENTOVER ROW	4	12,10,8,8	Supersets
PULLUP	3	To failure	Supersets
—superset with—			
DUMBBELL INCLINE PRESS	3	12,8,8	Supersets
CABLE CROSSOVER	2	12	Supersets
—superset with—			
SEATED CABLE ROW	2	12	Supersets
HANGING LEG RAISE	2	15	Supersets
—superset with—			
SITUP	2	20	Supersets
OBLIQUE CRUNCH	2	15 each side	

WEDNESDAY: THIGHS, CALVES, ABS

EXERCISE	SETS	REPS	ADVANCED TECHNIQUE
SQUAT	4	15,12,10,8	
WALKING LUNGE	3	12,10,10 each leg	
LEG EXTENSION	3	15,12,10[1]	Dropsets
ROMANIAN DEADLIFT	3	12,10,10	
LYING LEG CURL	2	12[1],10[1]	Partial reps
STANDING CALF RAISE	3	15	
WEIGHTED DECLINE CRUNCH	2	10	Supersets
—superset with—			
STRAIGHT-LEG CRUNCH	2	15	Supersets
HANGING OBLIQUE KNEE RAISE	2	12 each side	

FRIDAY: SHOULDERS, TRAPS, ARMS, ABS

EXERCISE	SETS	REPS	ADVANCED TECHNIQUE
DUMBBELL OVERHEAD PRESS	3	15,10,8	
DUMBBELL LATERAL RAISE	2	10[1]	Dropsets
BENTOVER LATERAL RAISE	2	10[1]	Dropsets
DUMBBELL SHRUG	3	12,10,8	
CLOSE-GRIP BENCH PRESS	3	12,10,8	Supersets
—superset with—			
PUSHDOWN	3	10	Supersets
BARBELL CURL	3	12,10,10	Supersets
—superset with—			
DUMBBELL HAMMER CURL	3	10	Supersets
REVERSE CRUNCH	2	15	Supersets
—superset with—			
MACHINE CRUNCH	2	15	Supersets

[1] Apply advanced technique to the set(s) indicated.

This program isn't easy, nor is it supposed to be. To stay on track, keep your goal consistently and clearly in mind, whether it's to lose three inches off your midsection or to drop your body fat levels into the single digits. Identify your goal, take measurements of where you are today, and post that information in a conspicuous place—in your office, on the fridge, wherever you'll see it often. It also helps to hang a picture of yourself today next to a picture from a magazine of what you want to look like.

TRAINING PROGRAM

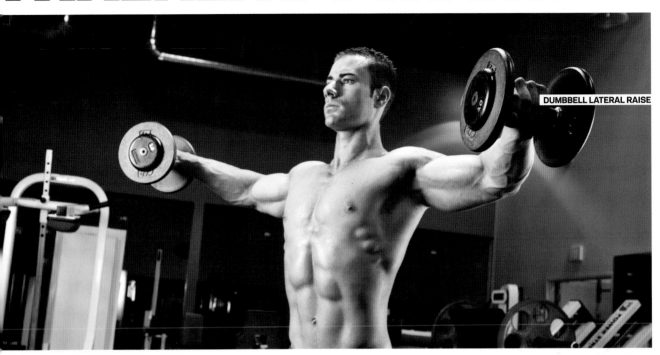

DUMBBELL LATERAL RAISE

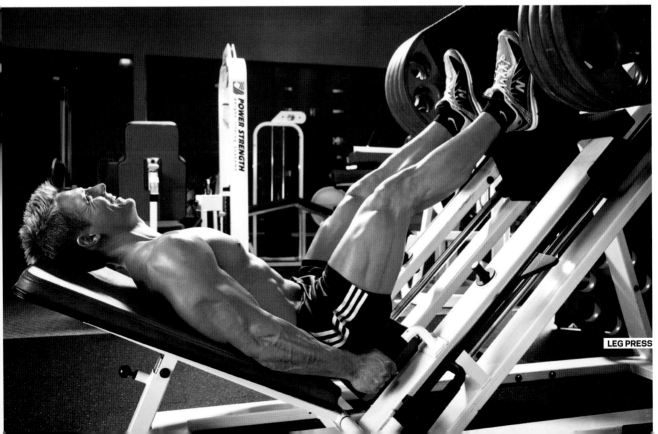

LEG PRESS

CARDIO COMPONENT

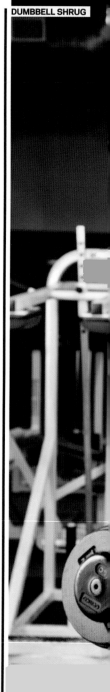

DUMBBELL SHRUG

THE HIGH-INTENSITY lifting you're doing will torch tons of body fat. To get as lean as possible, however, you need cardio. But it doesn't have to be boring. In Weeks 1–3, we recommend you do cardio four to five times per week; in Weeks 4 and 5, do cardio five to six times per week. Do it either after weight training or another time of day like first thing in the morning on an empty stomach. Each time you do cardio, choose any of the following five options:

INTERVAL TRAINING A
Equipment: Your choice of treadmill, elliptical, recumbent bike, or rower
Workout: Five-minute warmup; 25 minutes at a 1:1 ratio of high intensity:low intensity (like one minute of sprinting on a treadmill followed by a one-minute recovery jog); five-minute cooldown

INTERVAL TRAINING B
Equipment: Treadmill, elliptical, or outdoor track
Workout: Five-minute warmup; 25 minutes at a 1:2 ratio of high intensity:low intensity; five-minute cooldown

SPRINTS
Location: Indoor or outdoor track
Workout: Jog two laps as a warmup; 4x400-meter sprints with two minutes of walking between each sprint; jog two laps as a cooldown

LONG, STEADY-PACE CARDIO
Equipment: Treadmill, elliptical, or recumbent bike
Workout: Go at a challenging pace for 45–60 minutes; the pace should be difficult enough to break a sweat, but you should still be able to pass the "talk test" (where you can speak without becoming breathless)

HILL REPEATS
Location: Either on a treadmill at an incline or an outdoor hill (choose a steeper incline if you have a higher fitness level)
Workout: 10-minute jogging warmup; 10x50-yard sprints up an incline with one minute of walking recovery between each sprint (or a brisk walk/jog back down the hill); 10-minute flat-terrain jogging cooldown

THE WORKOUT—WEEKS 4 & 5

MONDAY & THURSDAY: LEGS, BACK, CALVES

EXERCISE	SETS	REPS	ADVANCED TECHNIQUE
LEG EXTENSION	3	12,10,10	Pre-exhaust
SMITH MACHINE SQUAT	3	12,10^1,10^1	Dropsets
LEG PRESS	3	10,10,8	
ROMANIAN DEADLIFT	3	12,10,10	
SEATED LEG CURL	3	12,8^1,8^1	Dropsets
PULLUP	3	To failure	
DUMBBELL ROW	3	12,10,8	
SEATED CABLE ROW	2	10^1	Dropsets
STANDING CALF RAISE	3	15	
SEATED CALF RAISE	2	15^1	Partial reps

TUESDAY & FRIDAY: CHEST, SHOULDERS, ARMS, ABS

EXERCISE	SETS	REPS	ADVANCED TECHNIQUE
BARBELL INCLINE PRESS	3	15,10^1,8^1	Forced reps
FLAT-BENCH DUMBBELL PRESS	3	10	
PEC-DECK FLYE	2	15^1	Partial reps
MACHINE OVERHEAD PRESS	3	15,10^1,8^1	Dropsets
CABLE LATERAL RAISE	2	10^1	Dropsets
REVERSE PEC-DECK FLYE	2	10	
WEIGHTED BENCH DIP	3	10,10^1,8^1	Dropsets
LYING TRICEPS EXTENSION	2	10	
BARBELL CURL	3	12,10,8	
EZ-BAR PREACHER CURL	2	12,10^1	Forced reps
HANGING KNEE RAISE	3	15	
CABLE CRUNCH	3	15	

1 Apply advanced technique to the set(s) indicated.

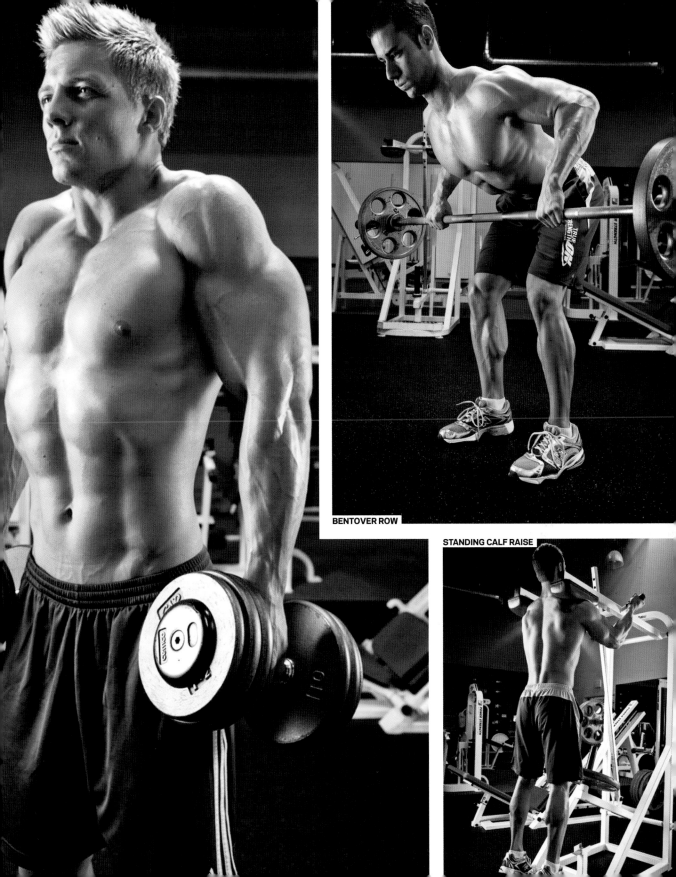

BENTOVER ROW

STANDING CALF RAISE

CHAPTER 5

FULFILL YOUR DENSITY

BUILD MUSCLE AND BURN BODY FAT IN LESS TIME WITH THE INNOVATIVE EDT SYSTEM

WANT TO DO SOMETHING REALLY DIFFERENT FROM WHAT YOU'VE DONE IN THE PAST? Something that won't take as long as those endless 30-to-40-set, train-to-failure-at-all-costs marathon sessions, yet will still make you bigger and leaner? The workouts in this new program won't hurt as much as your standard forced reps, dropsets, and rest-pauses, but you'll still train with plenty of intensity. In fact, experiencing less pain is kind of the point of escalating density training (EDT), a program created by renowned strength coach Charles Staley, B.S., M.S.S., director of Staley Training Systems in Gilbert, AZ (*staleytraining.com*).

"A lot of people assess the value or productivity of a training session based on how much it hurts, and that's a mistake," Staley says. "Fitness is a result of what you do, not what you feel. The focus should be on the amount and quality of work accomplished. When you do EDT workouts, you'll probably be hurting, but pain isn't the goal. If you're sore the next day, that's just because you're emphasizing performance over pain."

Confused? Don't worry, it'll make sense soon. Here's how it works.

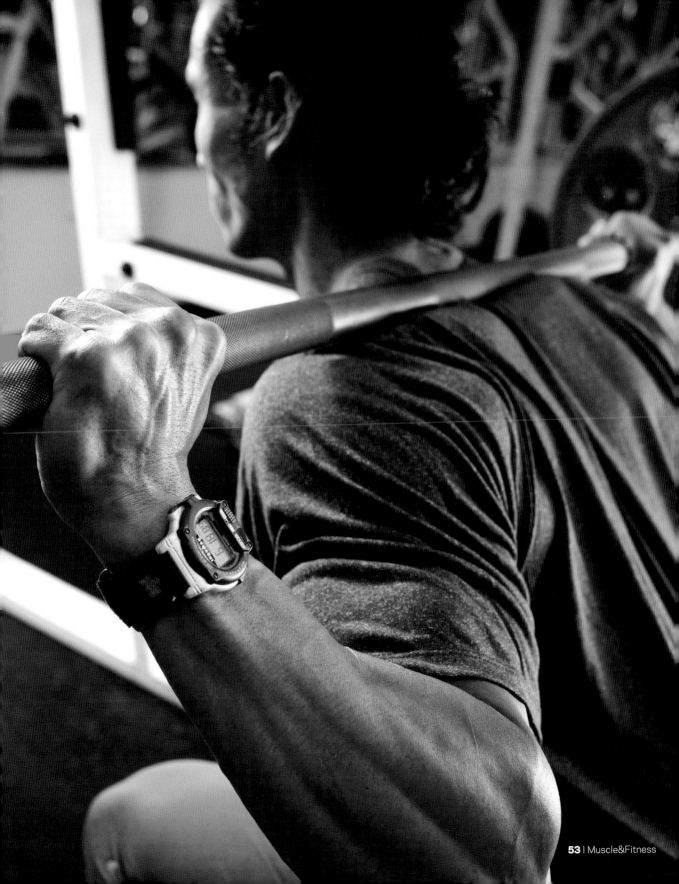

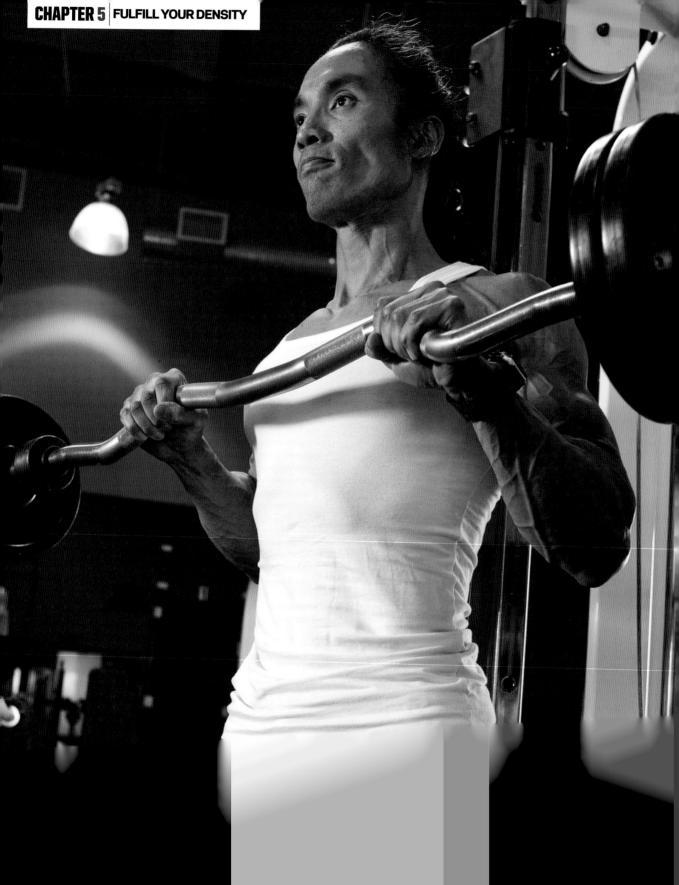

WHAT EDT IS

You select two exercises for opposing muscle groups (such as chest/back or legs/shoulders) and alternate sets between the two for 15 minutes. That's one PR (personal record) zone. Note how much weight you used and how many reps you performed for each exercise, and try to improve those numbers about a week later when you pair the same two exercises again. This helps you quantify how much work you've done. If the next time out you do more reps of each exercise with the same weight in the same 15-minute period, you've set a new PR and the workout was a success. EDT workouts are measurable and objective, and that's a good thing.

WHAT EDT IS NOT

EDT isn't about training to failure, at least not until the very end of a PR zone. If you select a weight for an exercise that's your 10-rep max (10RM), for example, you'll do no more than five reps at a time. Early on in the 15 minutes of an EDT session, this will have you stopping well short of failure.
"If you pace yourself—which, in this case, means not going to failure—you'll be able to do more work, and a big component of hypertrophy is the mechanical work performed," Staley explains. "If you train to failure on the first set, you drastically limit how much work you can continue to do. That said, it's OK to train to failure at the end of a PR zone."
Also, early on during a PR zone, you might rest only 5–10 seconds between exercises, but as you near the 15-minute cutoff, those rest periods may reach one minute. "As fatigue accumulates, you'll want to throw some longer rest periods in there," Staley says. "Be sure your form is good throughout. The beauty of EDT is that you make your own decisions; you have to learn the best way to pace yourself."

WHAT IT DOES

EDT routines are designed to improve body composition—helping you build muscle and lose body fat via intense (if relatively brief) training sessions. EDT can also be used to get stronger; simply increase the resistance and decrease the reps. But can you really get bigger, stronger, and leaner in such a short time?
"There's no question," Staley says. "This system is all about altering body composition. EDT can make you bigger, leaner, and stronger; it works quickly; and although you're training hard, it's enjoyable because the workout is a competition with yourself. There's a cardio benefit as well."

DEADLIFT

HOW TO DO IT:
Here's how you'll perform each PR zone:

SELECT TWO EXERCISES from opposing muscle groups. They don't have to be exact antagonists such as chest/back, biceps/triceps, quads/hamstrings or abs/lower back; you can also pair legs and shoulders exercises or quads and bi's moves. What's important is that you make sure each exercise fatigues only one muscle group. If you paired an incline press with a military press, for example, your delts would get so fried that you probably couldn't complete the 15 minutes.

SELECT AN EQUIVALENT resistance for each exercise, from heavy (4RM) to moderate (10–12RM) to light (40+RM), depending on whether you want to focus on strength, size or endurance. Whatever resistance/RM you select, start off doing half that number of reps. For example, if you go with your 10RM on incline presses and lat pulldowns, begin with five reps of each.

START YOUR STOPWATCH. Using a 10RM on incline presses and pulldowns as an example, do five reps of inclines, rest as needed (which will be very brief early on), and then do five reps of pulldowns. Continue in this manner until five reps is too much, then drop to four reps of each exercise. When four reps becomes too difficult, drop to three, and so on. By the end of the PR zone, you may still be doing five reps or alternating exercises every rep. When your stopwatch hits 15 minutes, that PR zone is over. Record your weight and total reps. A typical PR zone might look like this: 6x5, 3x4, 3x3, 3x2, 2x1, for 59 total reps per exercise. That's your current PR for that exercise pairing.

ABOUT ONE WEEK LATER, do the same two exercises, using the same weight as before, and try to do more than 59 reps to set a new PR. It doesn't matter how you reach your new PR; you can do more sets of five early on or do more sets of three in the middle.

"There's no wrong or right way to do this," Staley says. "The end justifies the means, and I'm not terribly concerned with the sets and reps. The focus should be on how much work is accomplished during those 15 minutes."

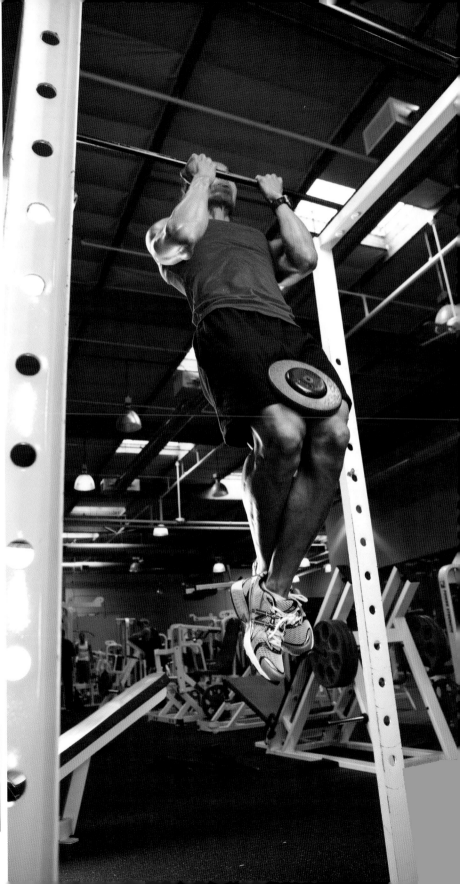

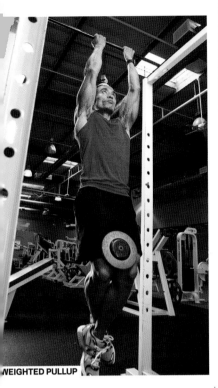

WEIGHTED PULLUP

HOW TO PROGRESS:

The point of EDT is to increase the amount of work you can do within a set period. In other words, it's all about making progress. Simply doing more reps with the same weight will allow you to progress, but soon enough you'll need (and want) to add weight. Staley has a simple formula for determining when to increase resistance: the 20/5 Rule. Once you exceed your baseline PR—the number of reps you did the first time you performed the exercise—by 20% or more, increase the load by 5% or 5 pounds, whichever is less. It might take you 2-3 repeats to be ready to increase the weight or you might want to up the resistance on your second go-around. Either way, once you add weight, you'll wipe the slate clean and build from there.

If you don't beat your PR, the 20/5 Rule works in reverse: If the number of reps performed is 20% less than your current PR, reduce your weight by 5% or 5 pounds (whichever is more) the next time out.

"Good performance, which is an indicator that you've fully recovered, is rewarded by heavier loads," Staley says. "Poor performance, however, means you haven't recovered, so you'll lift lighter loads as a form of active recovery. This reasoning runs counter to most people's intuition. But if you're weak, you need time to recover, not greater volume."

HOW OFTEN TO DO IT

To make significant improvements on your PRs, perform a given exercise pairing weekly for at least 3-4 weeks before changing the movements. But keep in mind: If you lift four days a week, you'll pair different exercises each workout. Let's say on Monday you paired incline presses and lat pulldowns. On Thursday you'd do chest and back again but with two different moves, perhaps dips and pullups. In this case, you'd do each exercise pairing only once a week.

HOW TO TWEAK EDT

There's a lot of flexibility in EDT, despite the finite lifting periods. But there's a reason each PR zone is only 15 minutes. "I believe more than that is excessive," Staley says. "I also believe in putting a time limit on your training. That's one of the best ways to get work done. But I'm not against people getting creative with my suggestions. If you want to experiment with longer or shorter PR zones or [more workouts per week], I'm fine with that. Just try it my way before you make any modifications."

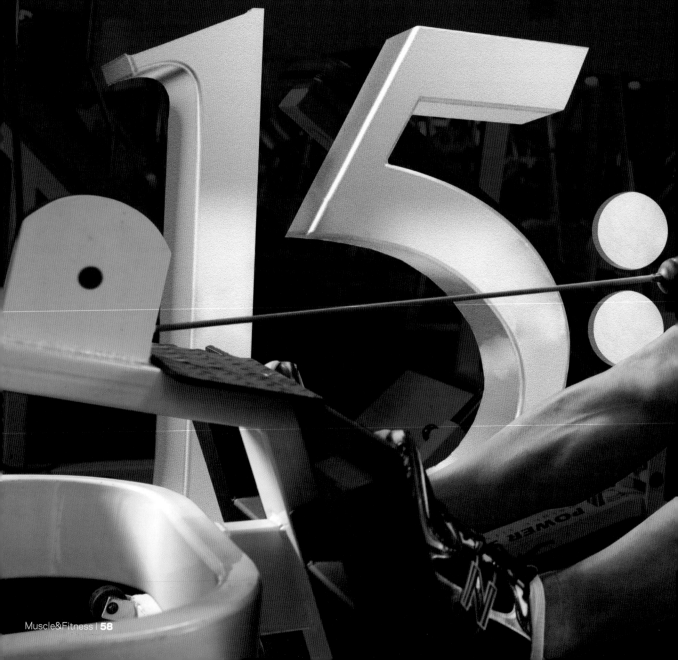

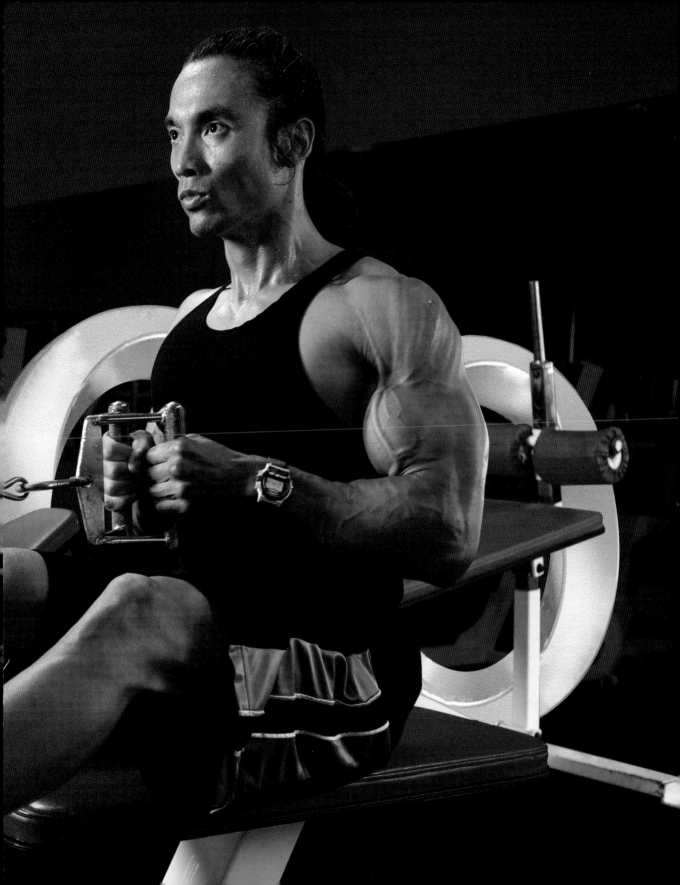

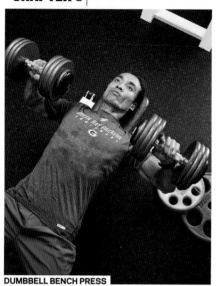
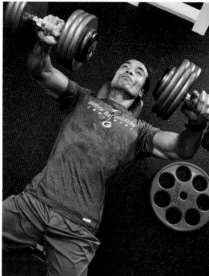
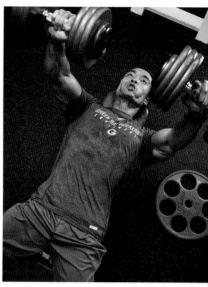

DUMBBELL BENCH PRESS

EDT PROGRAM

Below is a sample four-day-split, 12-week EDT plan. Within each four-week phase, exercise pairings (PR zones) are repeated once a week. Each workout includes one required ("compulsory") PR zone and one optional PR zone, each lasting 15 minutes, not including warmups. Whether you should complete the optional zone will depend on your training experience and fatigue level. Beginners should start with only the compulsory zone; advanced lifters can do both but should monitor fatigue levels and consider forgoing the optional zone if overtraining is evident.

The program is designed to work different body parts every four weeks to promote muscular balance and provide rest for potentially overstressed areas. For example, in Weeks 1–4, the shoulders are involved in every workout (chest/back and legs/shoulders PR zones), which could lead to overtraining. So direct shoulder work is minimized in Weeks 5–8, then reintroduced in Weeks 9–12.

>> For each PR zone, the resistance is listed in parentheses—from 6RM–20RM—to target size, strength, and endurance, and also enhance fat burning, over the course of 12 weeks. Always start with half the RM. When 10RM is indicated, start with five reps; when 20RM is indicated, reps start at 10.

>> Within each PR zone, alternate between the two exercises, resting as needed, until 15 minutes is up. Record the total reps performed for each exercise—that's your PR, which you'll attempt to beat next time out.

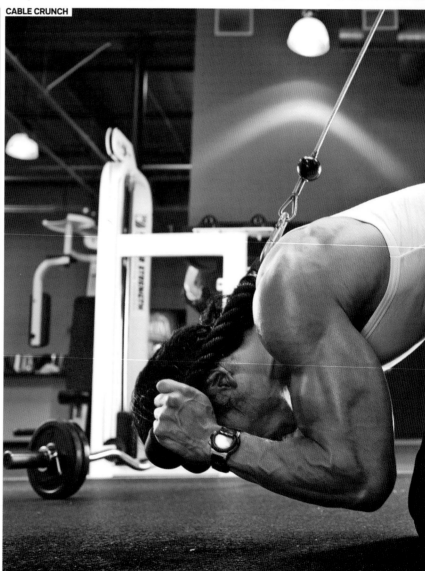

CABLE CRUNCH

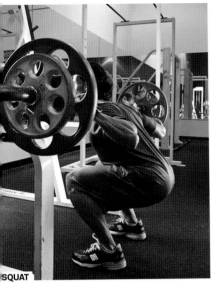
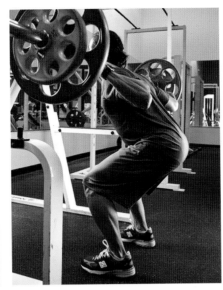
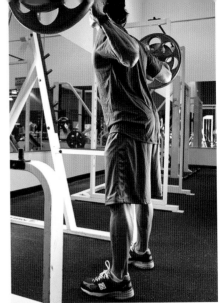

SQUAT

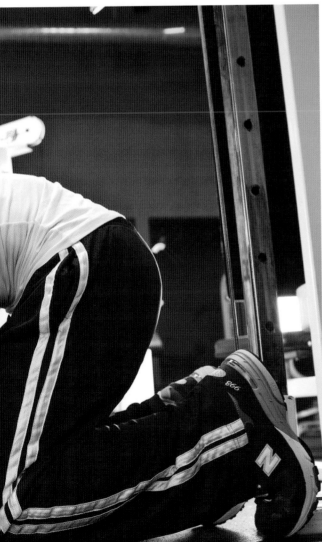

WEEKS 1-4

DAY 1
Compulsory: Dip/Pullup* (10RM)
Optional: Hammer Curl/Lying Triceps Extension (20RM)

DAY 2
Compulsory: Front Squat/Barbell Push-press (10RM)
Optional: Back Extension/Hanging Leg Raise (20RM)

DAY 3
Compulsory: Incline Dumbbell Press/Seated Cable Row (10RM)
Optional: Barbell Curl/Pushdown (20RM)

DAY 4
Compulsory: Deadlift/Dumbbell Front Raise (10RM)
Optional: Step-up (right leg)/Step-up (left leg) (20RM)

WEEKS 5-8

DAY 1
Compulsory: Front Squat/Seated Cable Row (10RM)
Optional: Standing Calf Raise/Barbell Shrug (20RM)

DAY 2
Compulsory: Dumbbell Bench Press/Hammer Curl (10RM)
Optional: Lying Triceps Extension/Reverse Curl (20RM)

DAY 3
Compulsory: Deadlift/Chin (10RM)
Optional: Exercise Ball Crunch/Lateral Raise (20RM)

DAY 4
Compulsory: Dip/Barbell Curl (10RM)
Optional: Back Extension/Pushup (20RM)

WEEKS 9-12

DAY 1
Compulsory: Chin/Front Squat (6RM)
Optional: Hammer Curl/Standing Calf Raise (16RM)

DAY 2
Compulsory: Dumbbell Overhead Press/Seated Cable Row (10RM)
Optional: Reverse Curl/Cable Crunch (16RM)

DAY 3
Compulsory: Dumbbell Bench Press/Squat (10RM)
Optional: Dumbbell Lying Triceps Extension/Barbell Shrug (16RM)

DAY 4
Compulsory: Pullup/Pushup (8RM)
Optional: Lunge (right leg)/Lunge (left leg) (12RM)

*If you can do more than 10 reps of dips or pullups, add weight; if you can't do 10 dips or pullups, use an assisted dip/pullup machine.

CHAPTER 6

SIZZLE YOUR FAT AWAY WITH HIGH-FREQUENCY TRAINING THAT HITS EACH BODY PART MORE THAN ONCE A WEEK—A LOT MORE

FREQUENT FRYER

We're well into the 21st century, but when it comes to weight training, some people are still intent on following workout dogma from the '80s and '90s. The idea that you should train each body part only once a week is as prominent in gyms right now as it was when so-called experts first advanced the theory three decades ago.

This once-a-week strategy gained favor because it addressed the concern that gym rats weren't giving their bodies adequate recovery periods and were thus overtraining and getting injured. Unfortunately, this alarm cry wasn't based on solid research; it was simply the thoughts of a few worried voices in the fitness world. Being cautious is good. Being overcautious is bad. In this case, it led to a generation of lifters more concerned with getting the right amount of rest than the right amount of training.

So, while a once-per-week training frequency is convenient for your schedule, it may not be convenient for your progress. This holds especially true for athletes who have been training each body part once a week since Ronald Reagan was president. Just as it's important to change your training poundage, rep range, and exercise order from time to time to prevent stagnation, you should change up your training frequency. As the Weider Principle of muscle confusion states, this will shock your body, which can result in newfound growth.

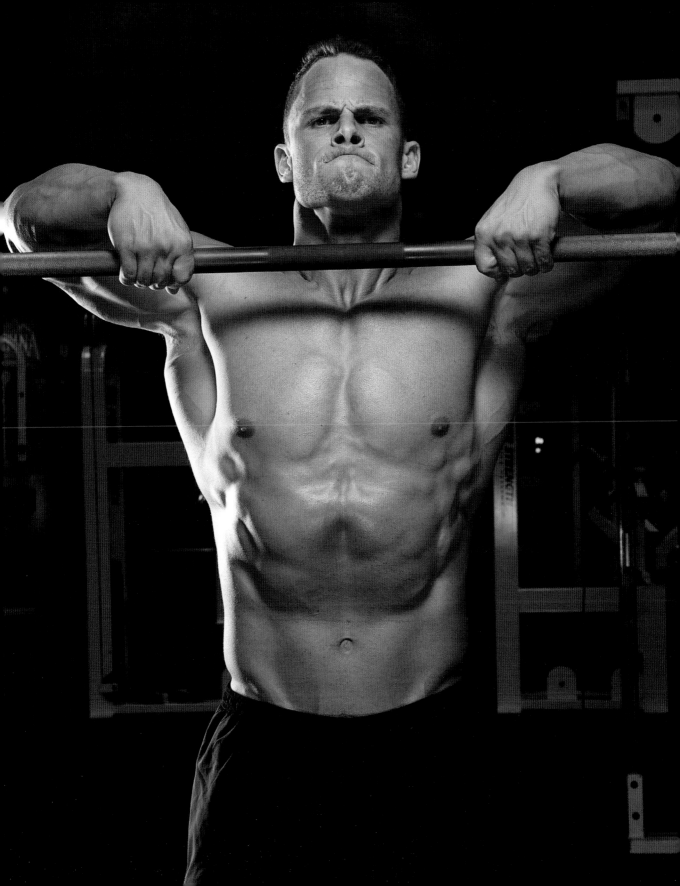

ROMANIAN DEADLIFT

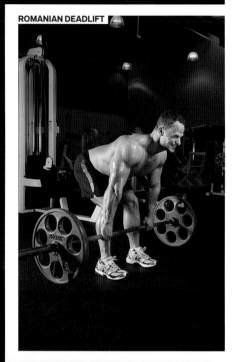

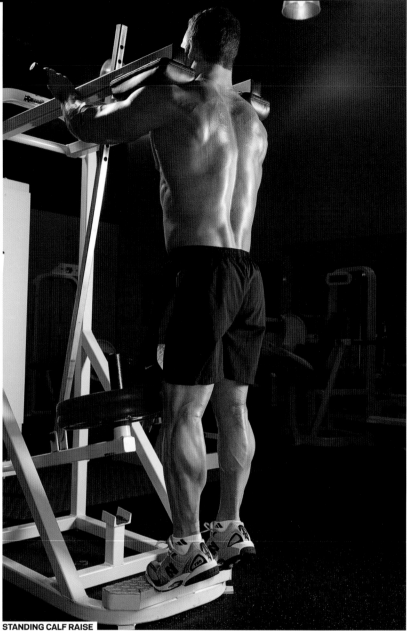

STANDING CALF RAISE

SUCH HYPERTROPHY is caused by the activation of genes in muscle fibers that are responsible for many of the adaptations that take place when you turn up your workout frequency. For example, consistent training activates certain genes that result in building muscle fiber protein, which means more size and strength. These genes are typically activated over hours, with some activated for even days. Repeated workouts, if timed appropriately, can build on the activation of those genes to reach an even greater activity level and, thus, increased muscle growth.

This is referred to as the staircase effect. In other words, let's say a certain gene involved in muscle growth is activated by a training session to the point that its activity is boosted by 100%, which slowly declines to 75% the day after the workout, 50% the second day, 25% the third day, and is finally back to the original level on the fourth day post-workout. If you performed the same routine on that fourth day or later, that gene would be bumped back up to 100% of its original activity. But if you trained on the second day, when the gene was still up by 50%, you could potentially bump its activity up to 150%. This is why training a body part every 48 hours could lead to even greater muscle growth and strength gains than training once a week.

Yet another way that more frequent training can improve your physique is that you have to train a greater amount of your body's muscle mass in each workout. With this program, for example, you'll train half of your body in one routine and the other half in the second routine. This is typically more muscle groups than you'd train in your normal split. Yet the more body parts you stimulate in a workout, the more growth hormone (GH) you tend to produce during and after it. GH levels during- and post-workout are now known to be critical for stimulating gains in growth and strength.

A higher training frequency also enhances fat burning through a number of mechanisms. First, training six days per week in which each workout trains half of the body means you burn a greater number of calories during and after training every day of the week. Training half of your body six times a week also keeps the genes and enzymes involved in fat burning ramped up. In addition, as discussed above, this program will boost GH levels higher, which is not only important for muscle growth but also aids fat burning by increasing lipolysis, the release of fat from fat cells.

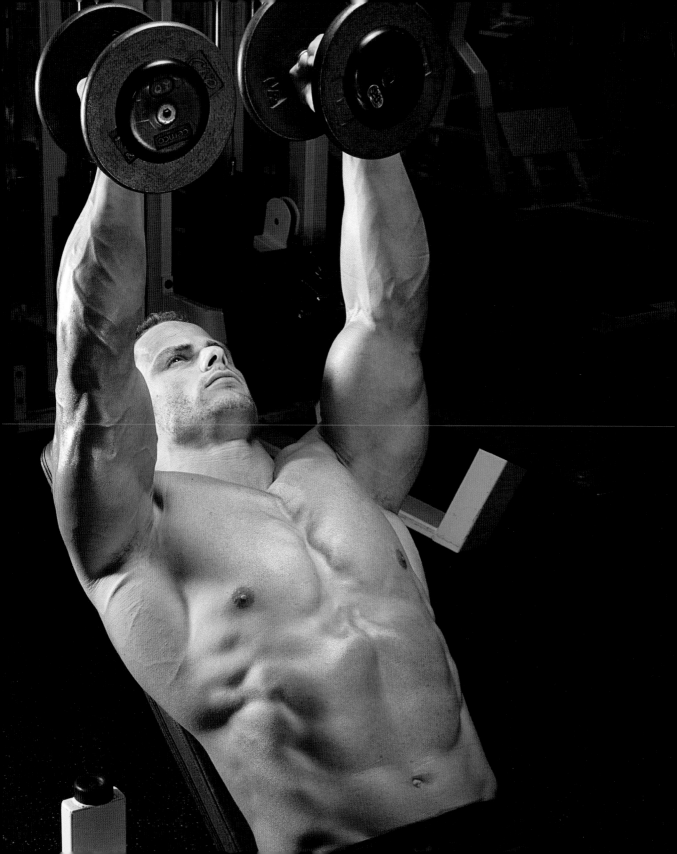

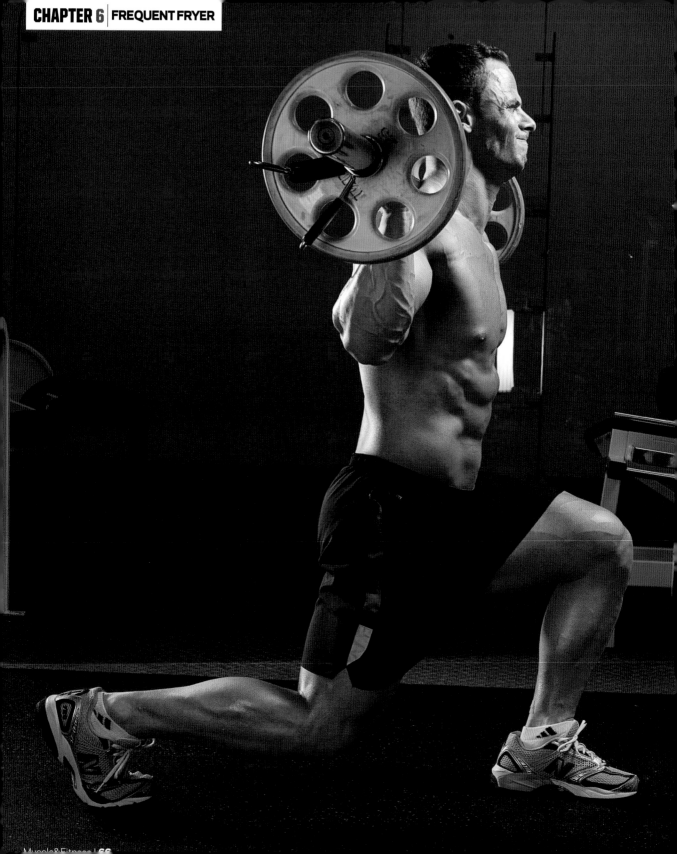

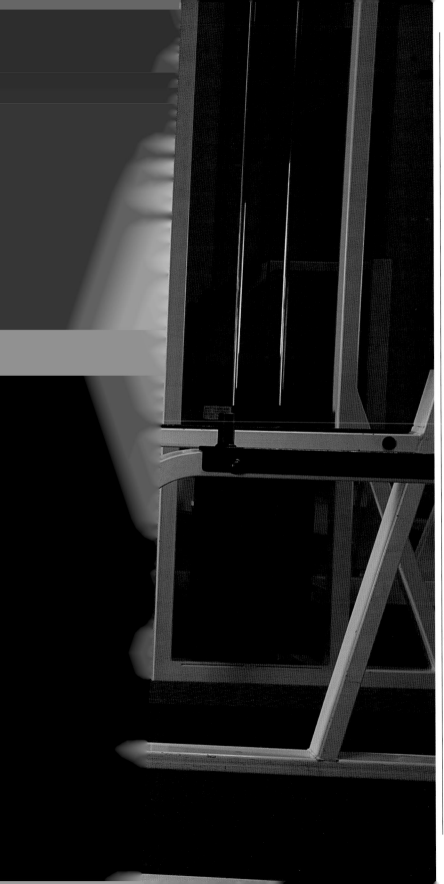

FREQ OUT

Our high-frequency plan has you follow a two-day split with half of your body trained in Workout 1 and the other half in Workout 2. The first routine hits chest, back, shoulders, traps, and abs, while the second hits quads, hams, calves, biceps, and triceps. These two workouts are repeated twice more during the week so that you hit every body part three times a week for a total of six workouts weekly.

Monday's workout, however, isn't the same as Wednesday's or Friday's. The three workouts you do each week for the same body part change dramatically each time in terms of exercises, weights, reps, and rest between sets. Varying the resistance and corresponding rep ranges builds strength, mass, and separation of the target muscles; and changing the rest time further enhances those adaptations.

Using chest as an example, on Monday you'll do the multijoint bench press and incline dumbbell press with a weight that limits you to six to eight reps with two minutes of rest between sets. This builds both strength and mass, and the generous rest time allows for maximal recovery so you can keep pushing heavy weight. Wednesday is isolation moves—incline dumbbell flye and cable crossover—and you'll drop the resistance to get 15–20 reps per set, decreasing your rest time to one minute to enhance GH levels and fat burning. On Friday you're back to multijoint exercises with the incline bench press and decline dumbbell press, but with a 10–12 rep range to focus on muscle growth; the 90 seconds of rest between sets will allow for greater recovery while still keeping GH levels high.

Doing two to three exercises per muscle group each workout for just six to eight reps may feel like undertraining, but we urge you to stick with the plan. After three workouts you'll total about 18–24 sets per body part each week, which is likely more sets per muscle group than you normally hit in seven days. Follow this program for four to six weeks, then go back to your regular training split and frequency. Return to this type of training frequency and split every four to six months to continue getting the gains you want.

M&F FREQUENT FRYER PROGRAM

MONDAY

EXERCISE	SETS/REPS	REST
CHEST		
Bench Press	4/6-8	2 min.
Incline Dumbbell Press	4/6-8	2 min.
BACK		
Straight-arm Lat Pulldown	4/15-20	1 min.
Seated Cable Row	4/15-20	1 min.
SHOULDERS		
Smith Machine Shoulder Press	4/10-12	90 sec.
Lateral Raise	4/10-12	90 sec.
TRAPS		
Dumbbell Shrug	4/10-12	90 sec.
ABS		
Rope Crunch	3/6-8	2 min.
Weighted Hanging Leg Raise	3/6-8	2 min.

TUESDAY

EXERCISE	SETS/REPS	REST
QUADS		
Squat	4/6-8	2 min.
Leg Extension	4/6-8	2 min.
HAMSTRINGS		
Romanian Deadlift	4/6-8	2 min.
TRICEPS		
Pressdown	3/10-12	90 sec.
Dumbbell Overhead Extension	3/10-12	90 sec.
BICEPS		
Cable Curl	3/15-20	1 min.
Concentration Curl	3/15-20	1 min.
CALVES		
Standing Calf Raise	3/6-8	2 min.
Leg-Press Calf Raise	3/6-8	2 min.

WEDNESDAY

EXERCISE	SETS/REPS	REST
CHEST		
Incline Flye	4/15-20	1 min.
Cable Crossover	4/15-20	1 min.
BACK		
One-arm Dumbbell Row	4/10-12	90 sec.
Wide-grip Lat Pulldown	4/10-12	90 sec.
SHOULDERS		
Barbell Overhead Press	4/6-8	2 min.
Upright Row	4/6-8	2 min.
TRAPS		
Barbell Shrug	4/6-8	2 min.
ABS		
Reverse Crunch	3/15-20	1 min.
Oblique Crunch	3/15-20	1 min.

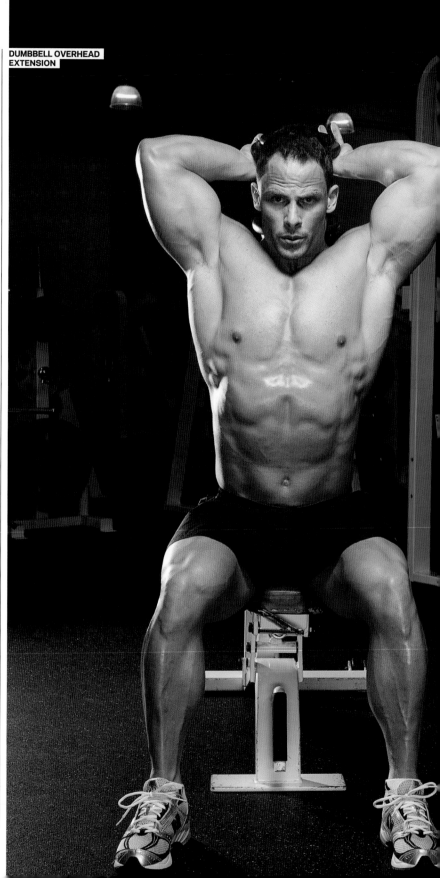

DUMBBELL OVERHEAD EXTENSION

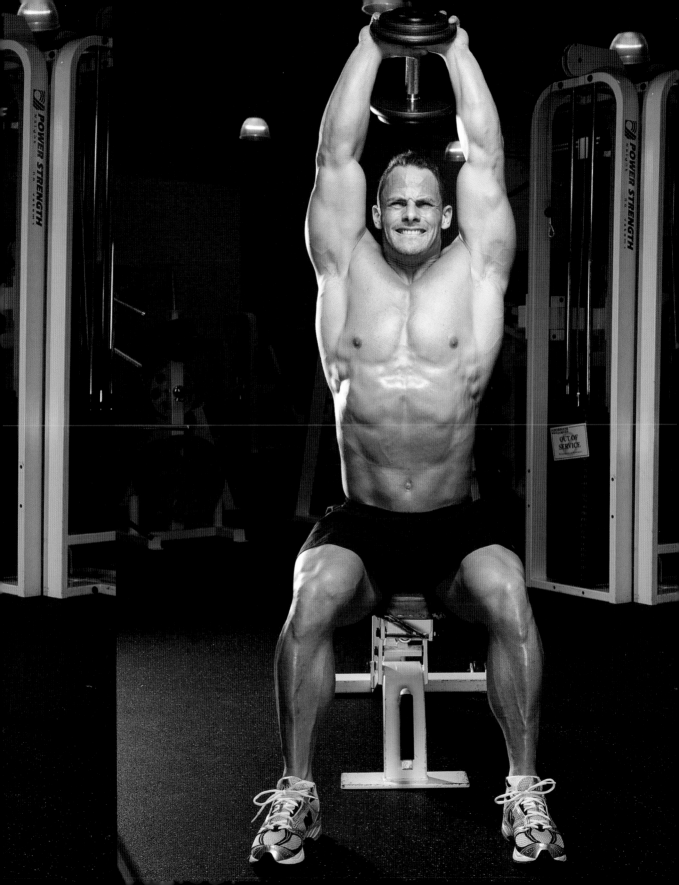

THURSDAY

EXERCISE	SETS/REPS	REST
QUADS		
Barbell Lunge	4/15-20	1 min.
Leg Extension	4/15-20	1 min.
HAMSTRINGS		
Lying Leg Curl	4/15-20	1 min.
TRICEPS		
Close-grip Bench Press	3/6-8	2 min.
Lying Triceps Extension	3/6-8	2 min.
BICEPS		
Preacher Curl	3/10-12	90 sec.
Incline Dumbbell Curl	3/10-12	90 sec.
CALVES		
Seated Calf Raise	3/15-20	1 min.
Standing Calf Raise	3/15-20	1 min.

FRIDAY

EXERCISE	SETS/REPS	REST
CHEST		
Incline Bench Press	4/10-12	90 sec.
Decline Dumbbell Press	4/10-12	90 sec.
BACK		
Barbell Row	4/6-8	2 min.
Reverse-grip Lat Pulldown	4/6-8	2 min.
SHOULDERS		
Cable Lateral Raise	4/15-20	1 min.
Rear-Delt Machine Traps	4/15-20	1 min.
Smith Machine Behind-the-back Shrug	4/15-20	1 min.
ABS		
Decline Crunch	3/10-12	90 sec.
Hanging Leg Raise	3/10-12	90 sec.

SATURDAY

EXERCISE	SETS/REPS	REST
QUADS		
Smith Machine Front Squat	4/10-12	90 sec.
Leg Press	4/10-12	90 sec.
HAMSTRINGS		
Seated or Lying Leg Curl	4/10-12	90 sec.
BICEPS		
Barbell Curl	3/6-8	2 min.
Alternating Hammer Curl	3/6-8	2 min.
TRICEPS		
Cable Overhead Extension	3/15-20	1 min.
Kickback	3/15-20	1 min.
CALVES		
Standing Calf Raise	3/10-12	90 sec.
Seated Calf Raise	3/10-12	90 sec.

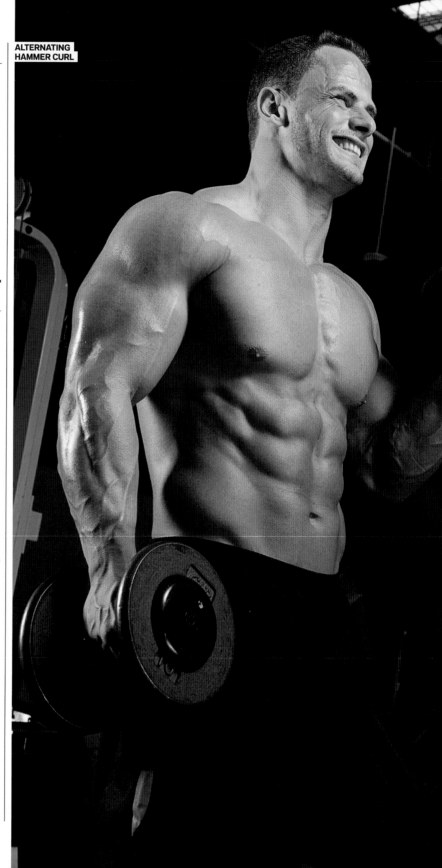

ALTERNATING HAMMER CURL

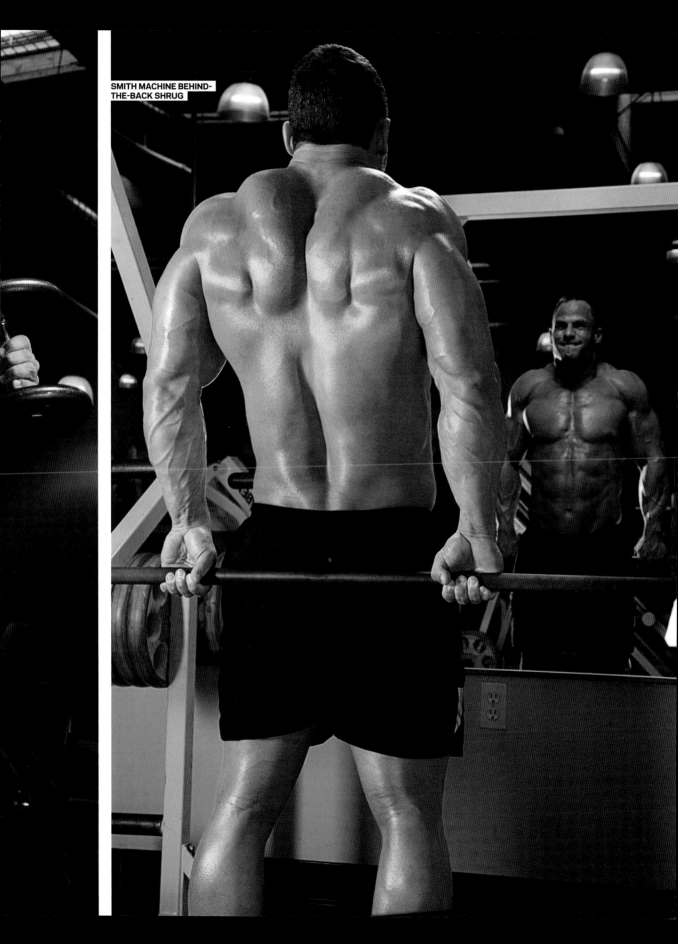

SMITH MACHINE BEHIND-THE-BACK SHRUG

CHAPTER 7

BURN FAT SAVE MUSCLE

GETTING SHREDDED FOR SUMMER CAN BE TROUBLESOME. THESE CARDIO AND NUTRITION TIPS SHOW YOU HOW TO STAY BIG WHILE GETTING LEAN.

You'd need a fancy calculator with an algorithm button to count the number of times "get ripped" has appeared on the pages of *Muscle & Fitness*. Its existence may seem mythical, but leaning out after a mass-gain phase isn't meaningless hyperbole. It may not be easy, but it is attainable. To do so, you need to target fat while preserving muscle.

In addition to dialing in your diet, you need a cardio plan: Not just endless aerobic exercise, but a program that fulfills the physiological needs of your body as it works on these two fronts. Consider our eight tips—a veritable muscle-sparing cardio blueprint—your very own guide to getting shredded.

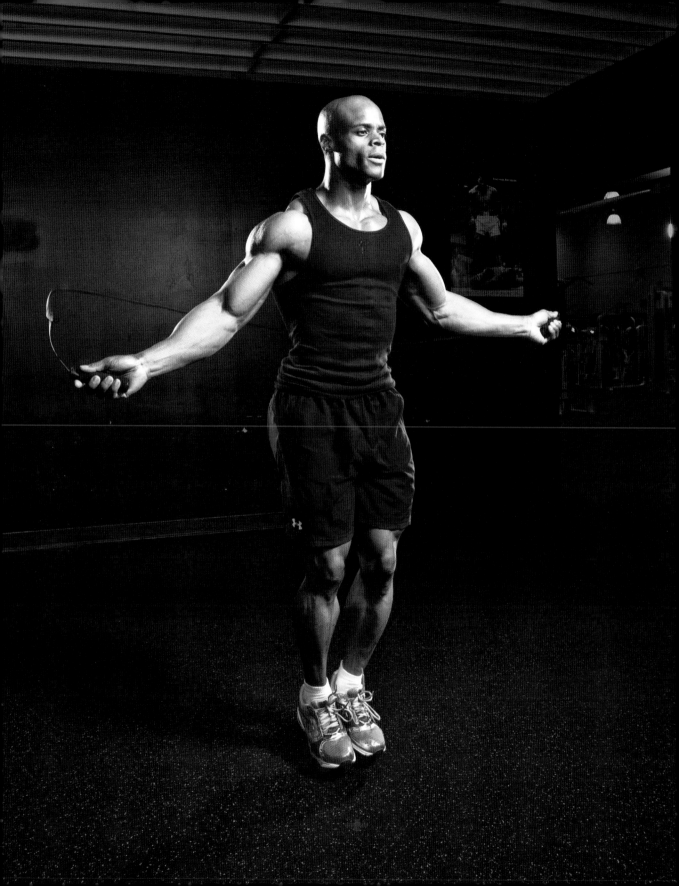

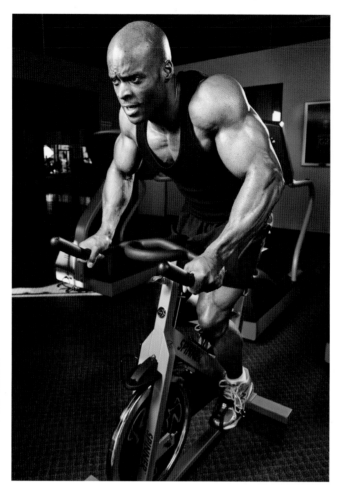

Shorter, more intense cardio sessions can be more effective than longer, steady-state workouts.

1 TIMING IS EVERYTHING

The temptation to do cardio before you weight train is understandable (and may, on occasion, be unavoidable). After all, if you're already warming up on a piece of equipment, why not knock out 30 minutes and be done with it? Answer: Performing intense cardio before lifting may deplete the body's stored glycogen, leaving little energy for weight training. A study published in the *Journal of Applied Physiology* found that decreases in blood-glucose concentrations can contribute to the release of hormones that break down muscle. In other words, training to build muscle while your body secretes catabolic hormones is a bit like using a strainer to bail water out of a sinking boat.

Doing cardio before lifting has also been found to blunt growth-hormone (GH) release. Japanese researchers found that subjects who did cardio before a weight workout experienced only one-third the GH response compared with subjects who didn't perform cardio first. In a subsequent study, subjects who did cardio after lifting weights also burned significantly more fat. This is because when you perform cardio immediately after weight training, your body must dip into body fat stores for energy because it has already used most of the stored glycogen during the lifting session. It also boosts GH levels, which can enhance fat loss and increase muscle growth.

2 THE POST-TRAINING CARDIO LIMIT

Keeping your post-workout cardio session to 30 minutes is important because you have a very short window of time after training in which to adequately restore glucose levels. By sticking to half an hour, you won't miss your opportunity to refuel and thereby prevent your body from entering a state of catabolism.

A short cardio session doesn't mean you're taking the easy way out, especially if you use high-intensity interval training (HIIT). Research has shown that much shorter HIIT workouts are more effective than the longer, steady-state variety. Australian researchers reported that subjects following a 20-minute HIIT program lost about six times more body fat than those doing 40 minutes of cardio at about 60% of their maximum heart rates.

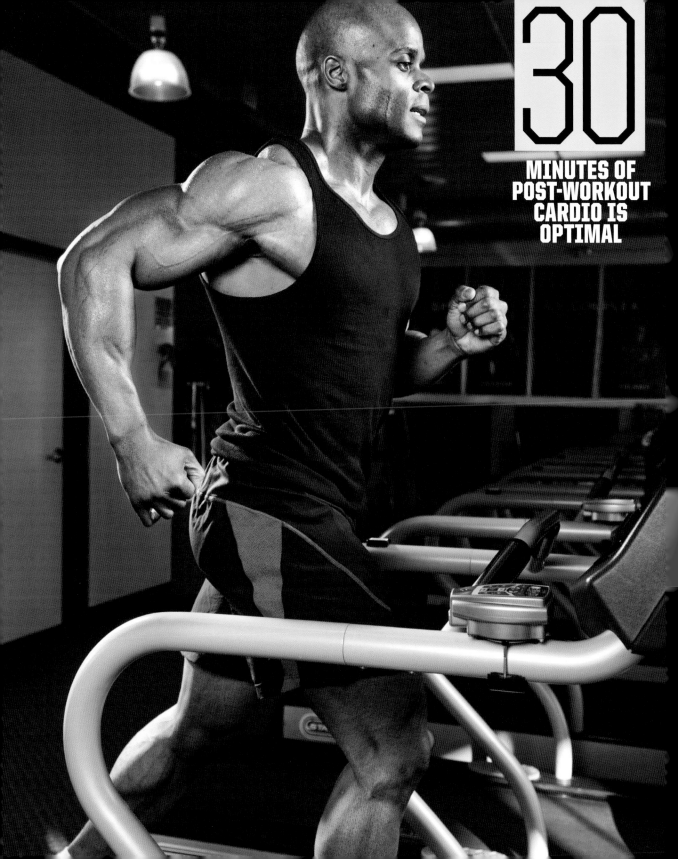

30
MINUTES OF POST-WORKOUT CARDIO IS OPTIMAL

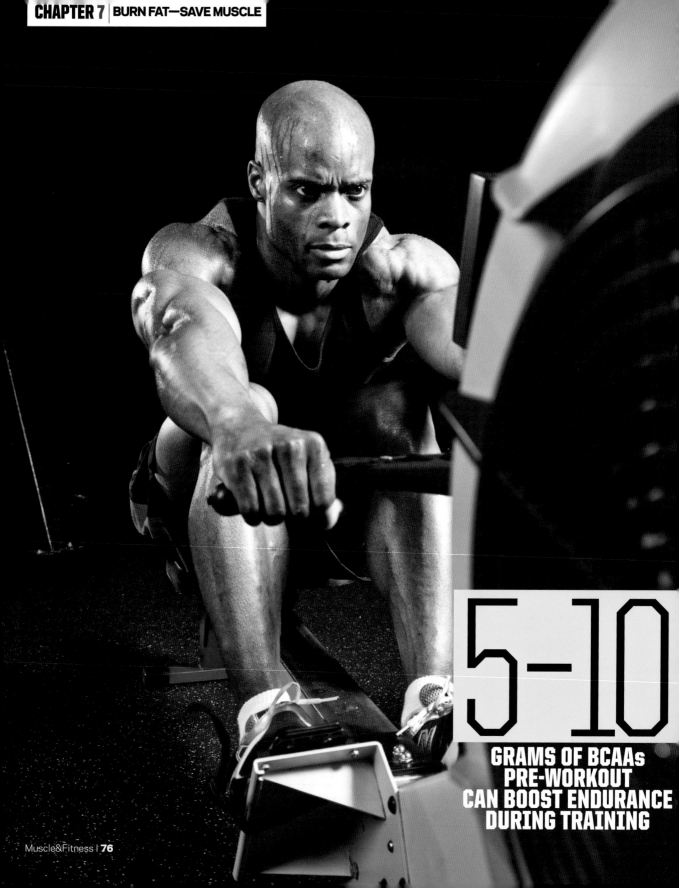

5-10

GRAMS OF BCAAs PRE-WORKOUT CAN BOOST ENDURANCE DURING TRAINING

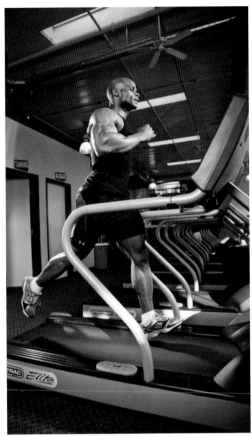

Unless it's unavoidable, save your cardio sessions for after weight training.

3 ALL AT ONCE, EAT

If you weight train and do cardio in the same session, don't do it on an empty stomach. Within 30 minutes pre-workout, take in 20-40 grams of slow-digesting carbohydrates and 20 grams of a fast-absorbing protein. Providing your body with nutrients that'll stay in your system throughout most of your gym session will help you perform at optimal levels and will prevent your body from digging in to muscle mass.

4 RICH & FAST

What about your weekend hikes and bike rides? They can last more than two hours (far longer than the recommended 30 minutes of cardio), so do you have to abandon them completely until you reach your get-ripped goal? You don't need to give up your outdoor fun, but you should provide your body with the proper fuel: 25-50 grams of high- and low-glycemic-index carbohydrates such as fruit and a sports drink or whole-wheat bread with jelly, and 10-20 grams of a fast-absorbing protein like whey protein isolate every 60-90 minutes to ensure your muscle isn't burned for fuel.

5 IN THE RED ZONE

Adequate testosterone and growth-hormone levels play key roles in keeping you anabolic and also increase your ability to shed body fat. In a study published in the *European Journal of Applied Physiology,* scientists had male athletes perform HIIT to exhaustion on a treadmill. Upon completion, subjects demonstrated a 38% increase in testosterone and a 2,000% increase in growth hormone. Try this interval program on for size:

BIKE
WARM UP 5 minutes (moderate intensity)
SPRINT 30 seconds (as hard as you can)
CRUISE 90 seconds (50% speed)
Repeat the cycle 10 more times for a total of 20 minutes
COOL DOWN 5 minutes (moderate intensity)

TREADMILL
WARM UP 5 minutes (moderate intensity)
WALK 1 minute at 3.2 mph at 12% incline
WALK 1 minute at 3.2 mph at 6% incline
Repeat the cycle 10 more times for a total of 20 minutes
COOL DOWN 5 minutes (moderate intensity)

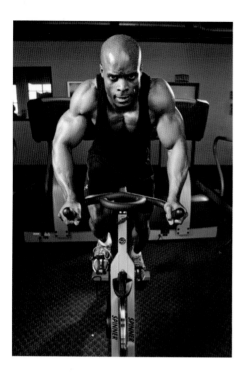

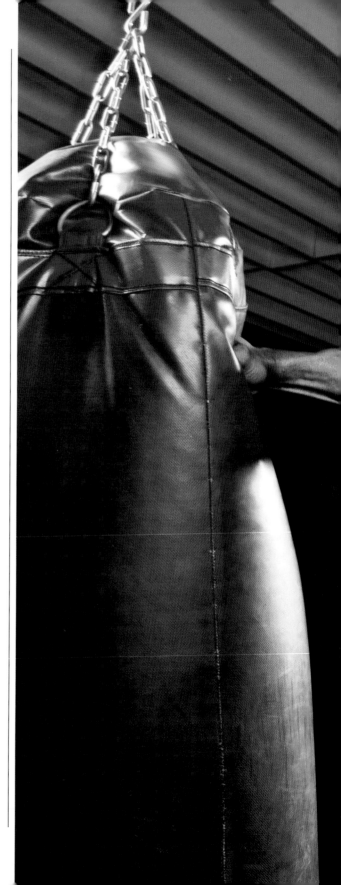

6 NOT QUITE EMPTY

When performing cardio first thing in the morning, do it on a relatively empty stomach. You'll have minimal glycogen stores from fasting all night, so your body must burn fat for energy. But you need to eat a little something to preserve your hard-earned muscle. Consume either 5–10 grams of BCAAs or half a scoop of whey protein beforehand. BCAAs are known to increase endurance during training as well as contribute to protein synthesis post-workout.

7 DIVIDE & CONQUER

If you feel you need more than 30 minutes of cardio a day, that's OK. Just limit each session to about half an hour. Cardiovascular exercise initially uses energy from blood glucose and stored muscle glycogen, but as training time increases and those sources of energy diminish, the body can switch to muscle for fuel. Keeping cardio sessions to 30 minutes will help prevent the body from cannibalizing muscle. Try doing half an hour first thing in the morning (after consuming your carbs and protein) and 30 minutes immediately after weight training.

8 ALWAYS REFUEL

The post-workout meal is more important than ever during a leaning-out phase. When your insulin levels increase and you take in a lot of aminos post-workout, the result is an environment made for muscle growth. Just make sure your macronutrient numbers are accurate.

Research suggests that casein be part of your post-workout nutrition regimen. After training, get 40–120 grams of fast-digesting carbs (a high-molecular-weight carbohydrate supplement, or white bread, potatoes, or rice) along with 40–50 grams of whey and casein.

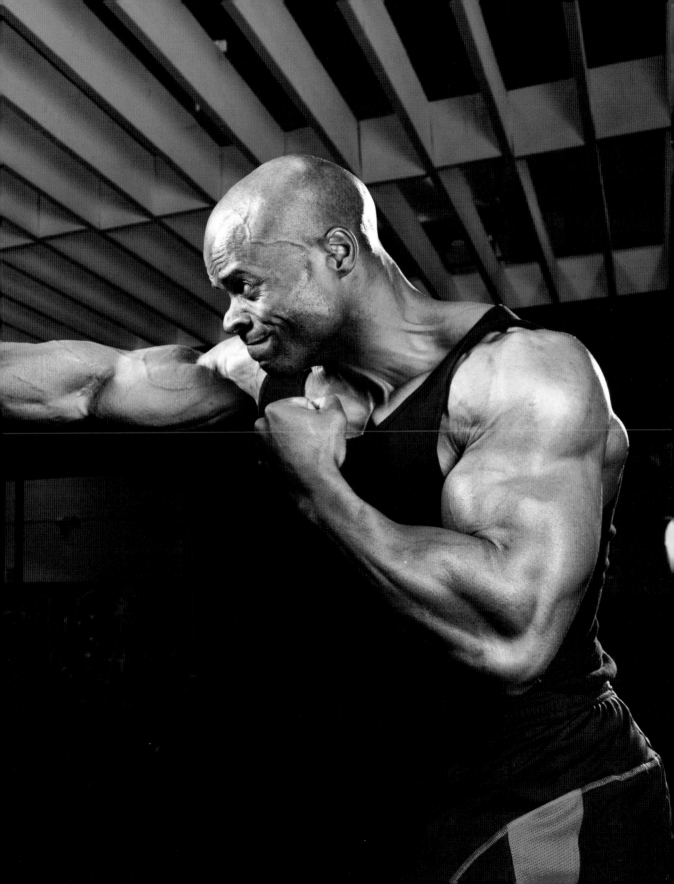

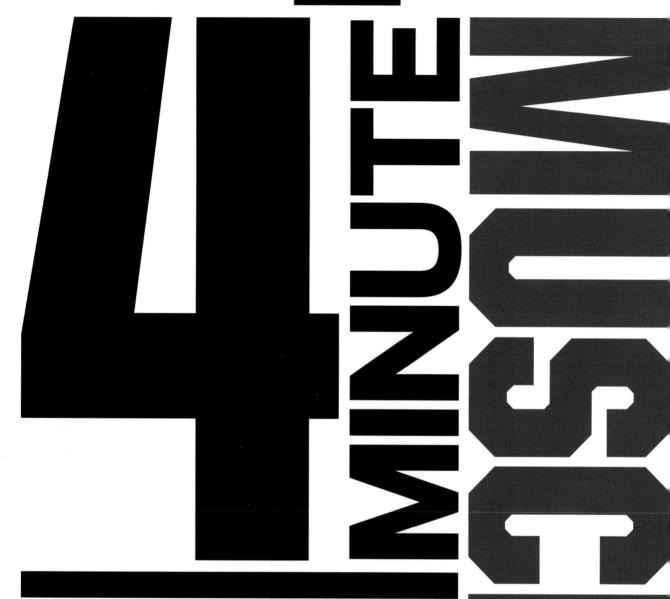

CHAPTER 8

4 MINUTE MUSCLE

PACK ON MASS AND BURN FAT WITH THESE BRUTAL TIMED SETS

What can you do with four minutes? If you put your mind to it, you can accomplish quite a bit. You could read several paragraphs of this article, run a mile if you're world class, or finish up matters with your girlfriend if you're young, virile, and in a hurry. But if you want to put on some mass and get stronger, our 4 Minute Muscle program will put your time-management skills to the ultimate test.

The concept behind 4 Minute Muscle is simple yet brutal in its execution. For each exercise in your workout, we want you to crank out as many reps as you can in four minutes. Then you move to another exercise for the same body part and do the same thing. This will fry your muscles in ways you've never experienced before while stimulating growth, burning fat, and getting you in the best shape of your life.

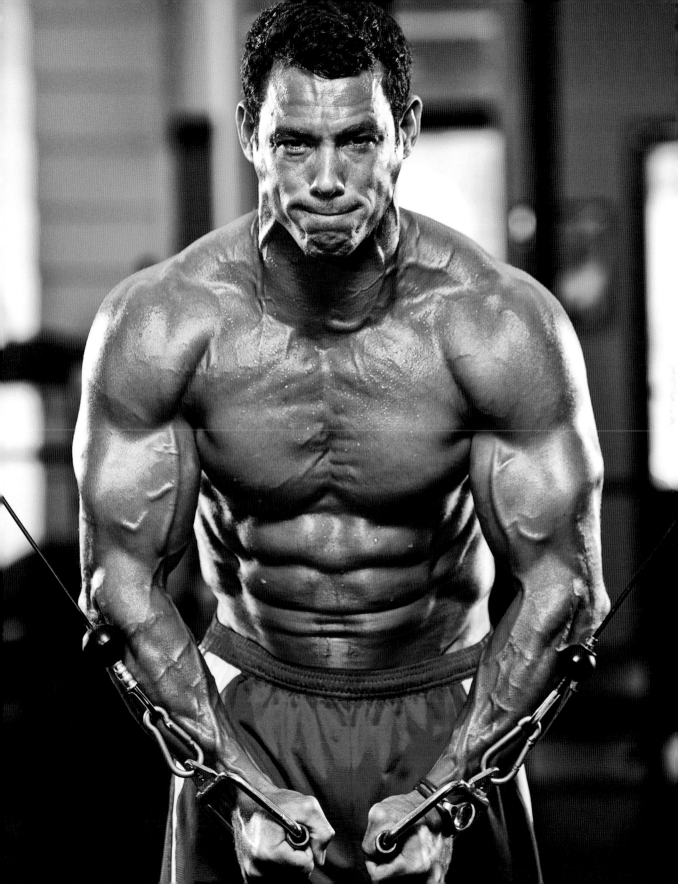

LONGER IS BETTER

Performing as many reps as you can in a certain period is an optimal way to train for muscular strength endurance. This is the ability to perform a task—in this case, moving fairly heavy loads in the gym—repeatedly for long durations with a minimal decrease in muscular efficiency. After following this program for six weeks, your failure threshold, the point at which you simply can't do another rep, will be significantly higher for each exercise.

Training this way improves your strength endurance because working your muscles to failure repeatedly puts them under a great deal of metabolic stress. This creates waste byproducts like lactic acid, which produces that "trapped in quicksand" feeling when you're about to reach failure. By intentionally training to create these waste products, you teach your body to better handle and dispose of them. That disposal process is how your strength endurance capacity increases. The better your body can do this, the longer you can perform a given movement. And the longer you can go, the more benefits you'll get from your workouts.

SIZE DOES MATTER

Strength endurance training, however, isn't designed solely to help you perform more reps. It also helps you pack on size by creating mechanical stress and causing muscle damage, both of which lead to rapid gains in muscular cross-section. This routine also instigates the release of anabolic hormones, the ones that repair your muscles and help them grow.

The program entails dramatically increasing both your training volume and the intensity with which you attack your workouts. Simply put, you'll train a lot harder than usual. As a result, you'll burn significantly more calories in each session and continue to burn them once you're finished. Combined with a sound nutritional program, this will strip fat from your body in record time. And since this is likely a drastic change from your typical training regimen, you'll experience the added benefit of shocking your muscles into growth. This is the Weider Principle of muscle confusion, and it works.

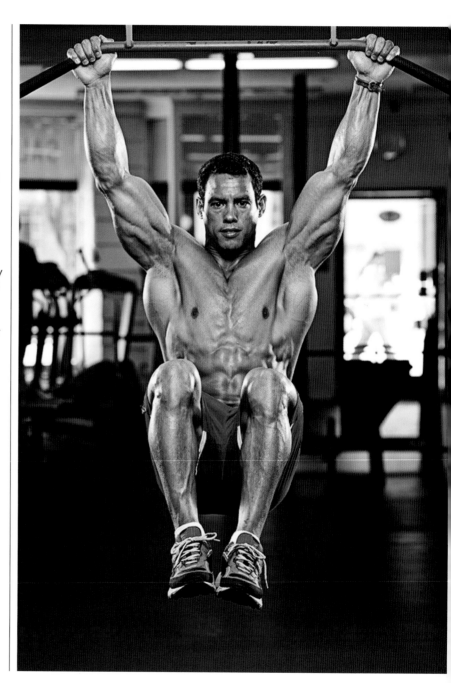

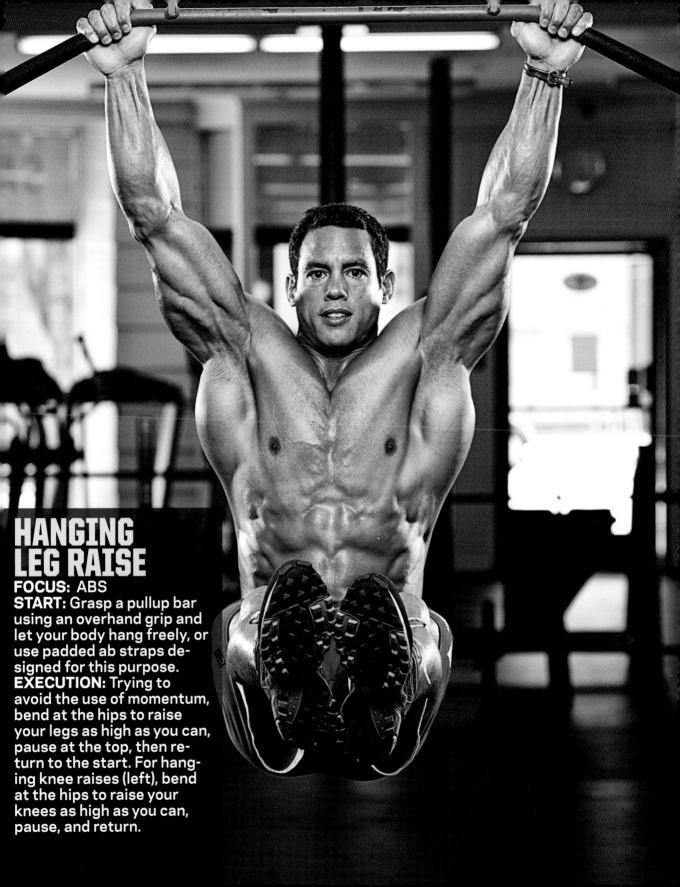

HANGING LEG RAISE

FOCUS: ABS
START: Grasp a pullup bar using an overhand grip and let your body hang freely, or use padded ab straps designed for this purpose.
EXECUTION: Trying to avoid the use of momentum, bend at the hips to raise your legs as high as you can, pause at the top, then return to the start. For hanging knee raises (left), bend at the hips to raise your knees as high as you can, pause, and return.

THE PREMISE

To get started, find weights with which you can perform 15–19 reps per exercise listed in the routines found later in this chapter. Follow the workouts in order, taking one preparatory week to establish and record the weights you'll use. Be accurate and stay within the 15–19-rep range because these are the weights you'll work with for the six-week period.

Your ultimate goal at the end of six weeks is to perform 60 reps per exercise in four minutes. The idea is to put in four minutes of total work on each move, taking a short rest period after reaching failure and then starting again. Weight selection is important because if you can't get at least 15 reps with a given weight, you won't even come close to 60 in six weeks, so it bears repeating that you must be precise here.

TIPS & TRICKS

There are two main ways to perform a 4 Minute Muscle exercise. The first way is how most people would intuitively try for 60 reps: by training to failure, resting, and then going to failure again, repeating this haphazard process until four minutes have elapsed. The primary drawback is that there are no systematic steps leading to an increase in the number of reps you can grind out. You're simply hoping your strength endurance will improve each time.

A far more intelligent strategy uses uniform rest periods between sets. For example, for the first two weeks of this program, rest for 20 seconds each time you hit failure. For the next two weeks, rest 15 seconds. For the last two weeks, take 10 seconds between sets. With rest periods that short, you'll have an excellent chance of hitting 60 total reps.

If you don't achieve this on every exercise, don't sweat it. We think you'll still be pleased with your results: bigger muscles, a drastic reduction in body fat, and the ability to perform significantly more reps with your usual weights on every move in the gym.

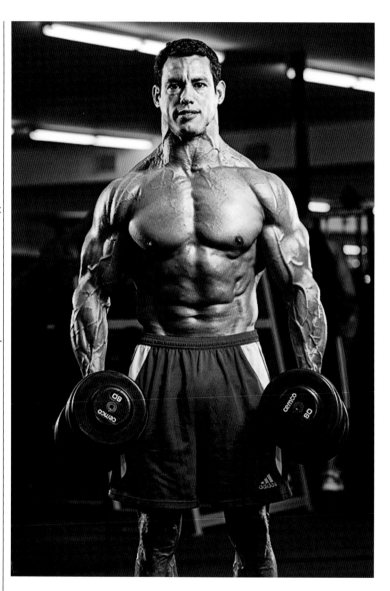

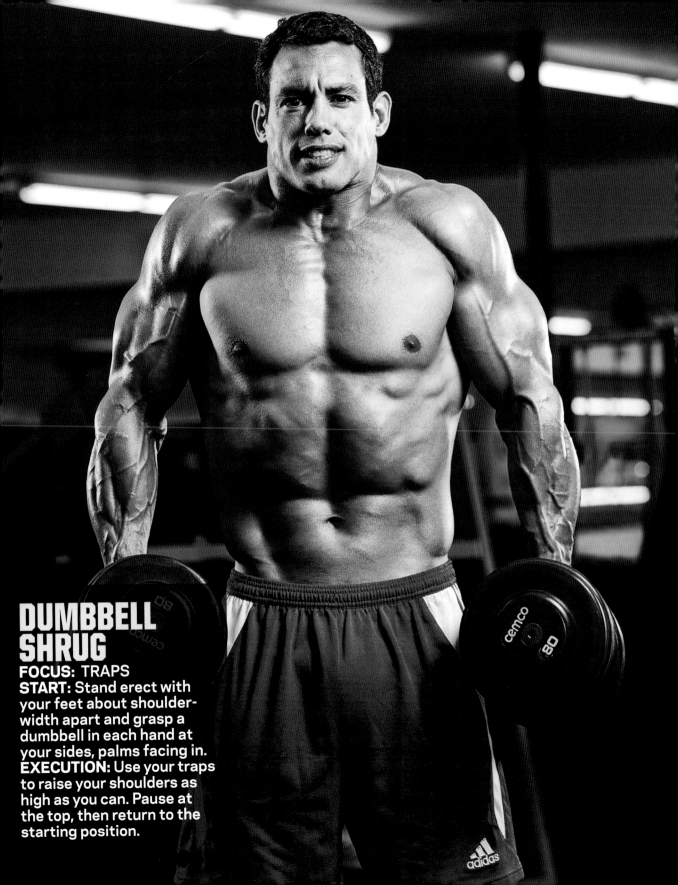

DUMBBELL SHRUG

FOCUS: TRAPS
START: Stand erect with your feet about shoulder-width apart and grasp a dumbbell in each hand at your sides, palms facing in.
EXECUTION: Use your traps to raise your shoulders as high as you can. Pause at the top, then return to the starting position.

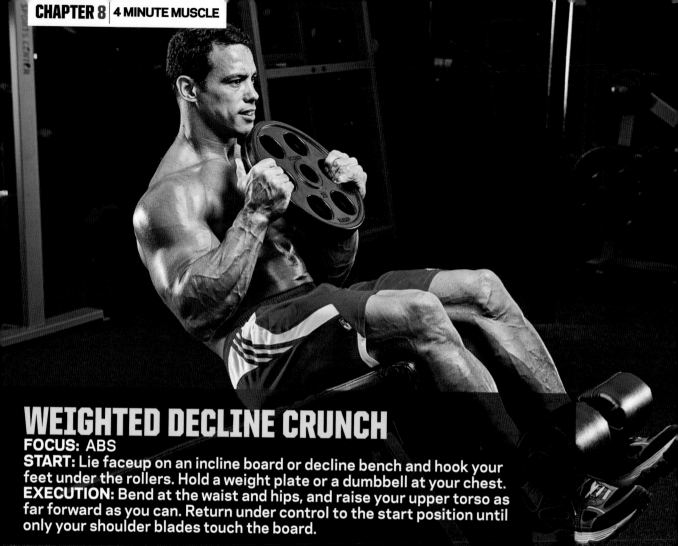

WEIGHTED DECLINE CRUNCH

FOCUS: ABS

START: Lie faceup on an incline board or decline bench and hook your feet under the rollers. Hold a weight plate or a dumbbell at your chest.

EXECUTION: Bend at the waist and hips, and raise your upper torso as far forward as you can. Return under control to the start position until only your shoulder blades touch the board.

4 MINUTE MUSCLE WORKOUTS

WORKOUT 1 (MONDAY)

Chest, Biceps, Abs

EXERCISE

Smith Machine Bench Press

Dumbbell Bench Press

Dumbbell Incline Flye

Cable Crossover

Barbell Curl

Dumbbell Incline Curl

Preacher Curl

Barbell Wrist Curl

Hanging Leg or Knee Raise[1]

Cable Crunch

WORKOUT 2 (WEDNESDAY)

Back, Triceps

EXERCISE

Wide-grip Lat Pulldown[2]

Seated Cable Row[2]

Reverse-grip Lat Pulldown[2]

Straight-arm Lat Pulldown

Smith Machine Close-grip Bench Press

Pushdown

Cable Overhead Triceps Extension

WORKOUT 3 (THURSDAY)

Shoulders, Traps

EXERCISE

Smith Machine Overhead Press

Dumbbell Lateral Raise

Dumbbell Overhead Press

Cable Bentover Lateral Raise

Smith Machine Shrug[2]

Dumbbell Shrug[2]

WORKOUT 4 (FRIDAY)

Legs, Abs

EXERCISE

Smith Machine Squat

Leg Press

Leg Extension

Romanian Deadlift[2]

Lying Leg Curl

Standing Calf Raise

Seated Calf Raise

Weighted Decline Crunch

Reverse Crunch

1 If you can't perform 15 reps with straight legs, bend your knees. If you can do more than 19 reps, hold a medicine ball or dumbbell between your feet or knees.

2 Use wrist straps for this exercise.

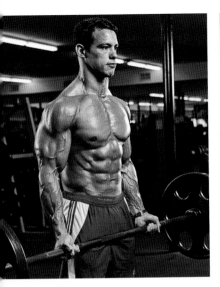

PUSHDOWN

FOCUS: TRICEPS

START: Attach a rope handle or bar to a high-pulley cable and stand erect facing the weight stack. Grasp the handle with both hands at about chest level.

EXECUTION: Push the handle down by extending your arms until your elbows are nearly locked out, then return under control to the start. Keep your elbows pinned to your sides.

DUMBBELL INCLINE FLYE

FOCUS: CHEST

START: Grasp two dumbbells and lie faceup on an incline bench. Hold the weights over your chest with your palms facing in and your elbows slightly bent.

EXECUTION: Maintaining the slight bend in your elbows, lower the dumbbells out to your sides until you feel a stretch in your pecs, then return to the start with the weights over your chest.

REVERSE CRUNCH

FOCUS: ABS

START: Lie faceup on the floor with your hips and knees bent 90 degrees so your lower legs are elevated and parallel to the floor. Keep your arms at your sides with your hands flat on the floor for support.

EXECUTION: Bend at the waist to bring your knees toward your chest. Return to the start position under control.

STRAIGHT-ARM LAT PULLDOWN

FOCUS: LATS

START: Attach a lat pulldown bar to a high-pulley cable, then stand erect and grasp the bar at the ends using an overhand grip.

EXECUTION: Keeping your arms straight, use your lats to pull the bar down until it touches your quads. Slowly return to the start position.

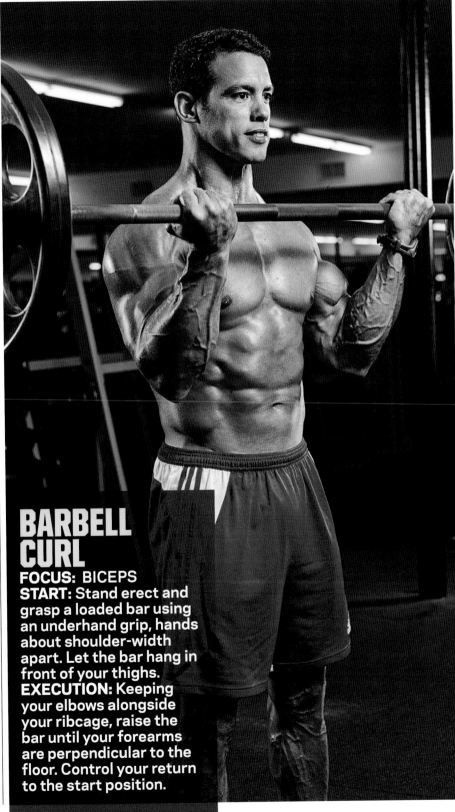

BARBELL CURL

FOCUS: BICEPS

START: Stand erect and grasp a loaded bar using an underhand grip, hands about shoulder-width apart. Let the bar hang in front of your thighs.

EXECUTION: Keeping your elbows alongside your ribcage, raise the bar until your forearms are perpendicular to the floor. Control your return to the start position.

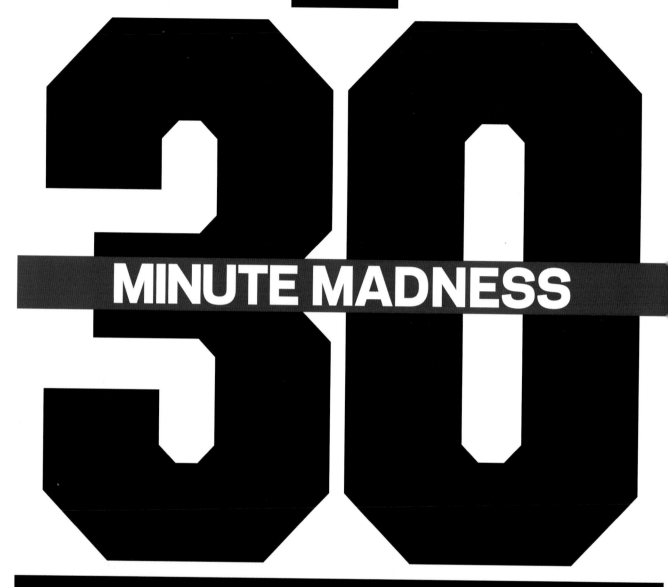

CHAPTER 9

30 MINUTE MADNESS

SAVE TIME AND GET LEAN WITH THESE 10 BRUTAL WORKOUTS THAT WILL TORCH BODY FAT IN 30 MINUTES OR LESS

It's like poison to your ears: Get your workout done in just 30 minutes or less. It sounds like an infomercial gimmick that has no place in your life or in this magazine, but nothing could be further from the truth. A properly designed half-hour training session can pack just as much of a punch as a standard 60-minute workout—if not more. That's good news, because no matter how dedicated you are to your training, December has a way of leeching time out of your life and funneling it into all kinds of crap you'd rather not be bothered with. No matter what type of program you're following, we've got you covered with one of these 10 workouts that, yes, take 30 minutes or less to complete. The trainers who designed them are some of the most highly regarded and highly sought-after names in the industry. They also walk the walk themselves. Full-time jobs and heavy client loads often leave them just 30 minutes to train—and they still get the job done.

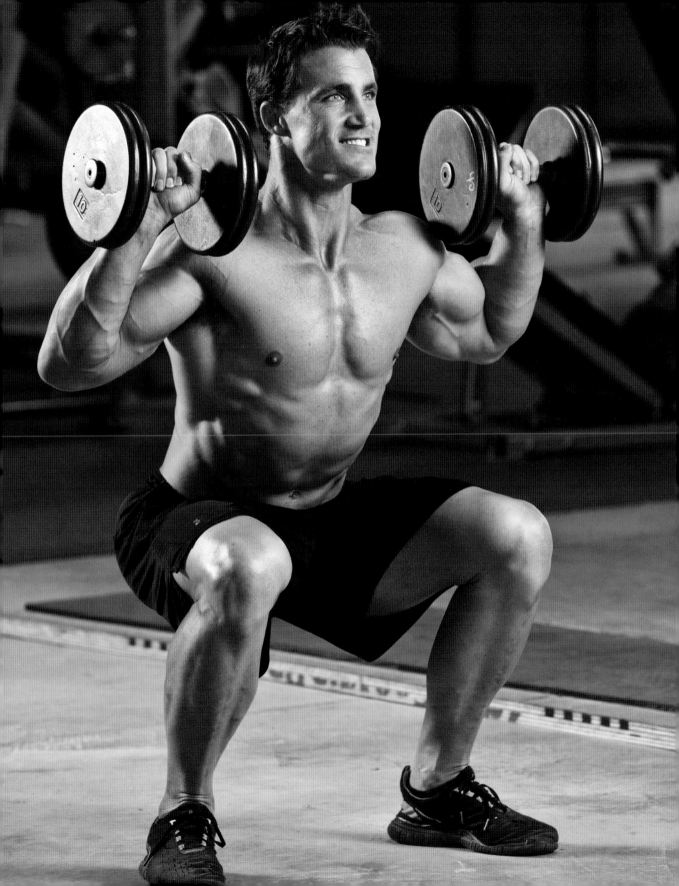

WHAT'S HERE

If you follow a body-part split, we've provided four separate routines for your legs, chest, and back; bi's and tri's; and shoulders and traps. The volume is high, rest is short, and you won't stop moving from station to station. Best of all, you're going to get the kind of pump you've come to expect from a one-hour session. If you don't fit neatly into the body-part split category, there are six total-body programs to choose from to keep all your muscles working hard and your conditioning levels high. You can rotate them and attack three or four per week, or you can simply use one as a stop-gap when there's no time for your regular program. There's challenge, variety, and plenty of time saved.

But there's one thing you won't find here: Excuses.

DB ROMANIAN DEADLIFT TO UPRIGHT ROW [WORKOUT 5] Hold two dumbbells and stand in a shoulder-width stance. Push your hips back and lower the weights to the middle of your shins. Engage your hamstrings to stand up, then row the dumbbells to shoulder level.

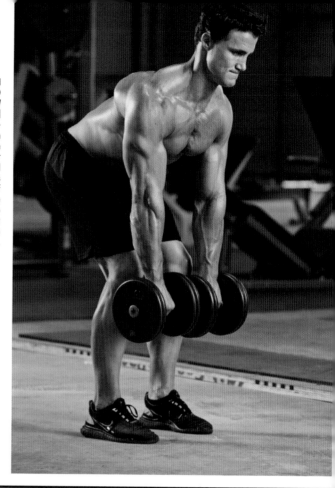

1

THREE-HEADED MONSTER
TARGET: TOTAL BODY

THE IDEA: *Eight exercises—all compound movements—performed in a straight circuit, three times through. Hit 8–12 reps of each exercise. Rest only as long as is necessary to get to the next station and only 60–90 seconds at the end of each circuit.*

THE WORKOUT:

Back Squat
Pullup
Walking Lunge
Pushup
Bulgarian Split Squat
DB Squat to Press
Hanging Knee Raise
Situp

Trainer: Harry Selkow

2

THE SLEEVE BUSTER
TARGET: SHOULDERS AND TRAPS

THE IDEA: *Time constraints leave you with only 20–30 seconds to rest between exercises if you want to achieve the necessary volume. Failure lurks behind every rep, so make sure you work with a spotter or at least the spotter bars of a power rack. After the barbell military press, the rest of the workout focuses on the lateral and rear heads of the deltoid, as well as the muscles surrounding your shoulders (triceps and back). Work 3A and 3B, and 4A and 4B, as supersets.*

THE WORKOUT:

Warmup: 30 Body-weight Squats & 10 Burpees

1) Barbell Military Press: 1x12, 3xAMAP*
2) Close-grip Bench Press: 1x12, 3xAMAP
3A) Pullup: 3x8
3B) Rear Delt Flye: 3x12
4A) DB Scaption: 3x12
4B) Face Pull: 3x15

*As many as possible
Trainer: Jim Smith

3

GET THE BUCKET
TARGET: TOTAL BODY

THE IDEA: *Rest is for the weak. You can get an hour-plus of volume in half the time as long as you stay focused and choose sensible weights. All your work is broken into three mini-circuits. Finish everything in one circuit before moving on to the next. But be warned: Even while using weights you can manage without breaking form, there are 30 total sets here, meaning you have to average one set per minute to finish on time.*

THE WORKOUT:

1A) Front Squat: 10,9,8
1B) DB Flat Bench: 3x10
1C) Single-arm Medicine Ball Slam: 3x8 each side
1D) DB Scaption: 3x12
2A) DB Romanian Deadlift: 3x8
2B) Inverted Row: 3x10
2C) Military Press: 3x10
3A) DB Kickback: 3x10
3B) Barbell Curl: 3x10
3C) Swiss Ball Leg Curl: 3x12

Trainer: Brian Thompson

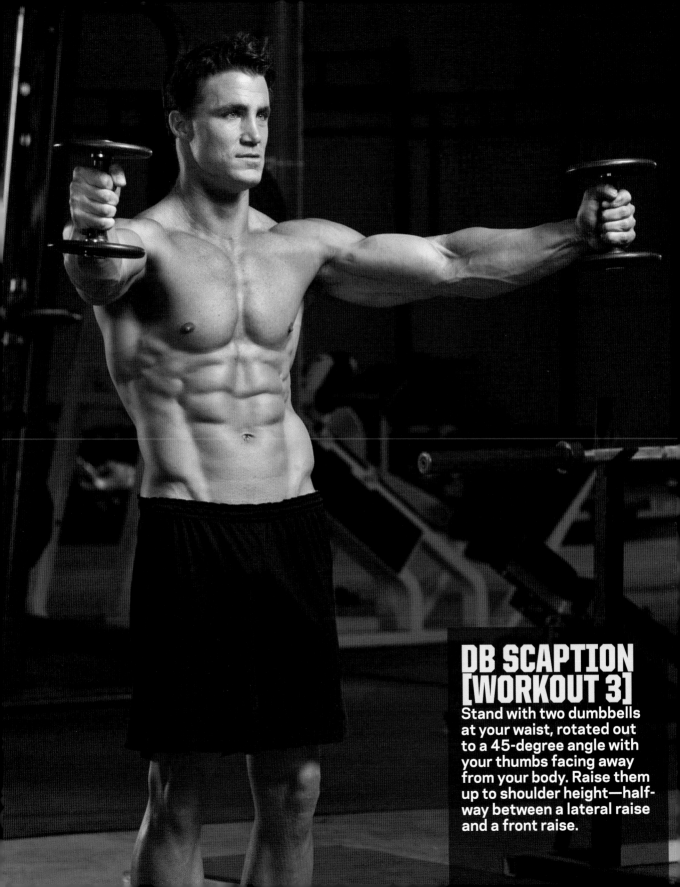

DB SCAPTION
[WORKOUT 3]

Stand with two dumbbells at your waist, rotated out to a 45-degree angle with your thumbs facing away from your body. Raise them up to shoulder height—half-way between a lateral raise and a front raise.

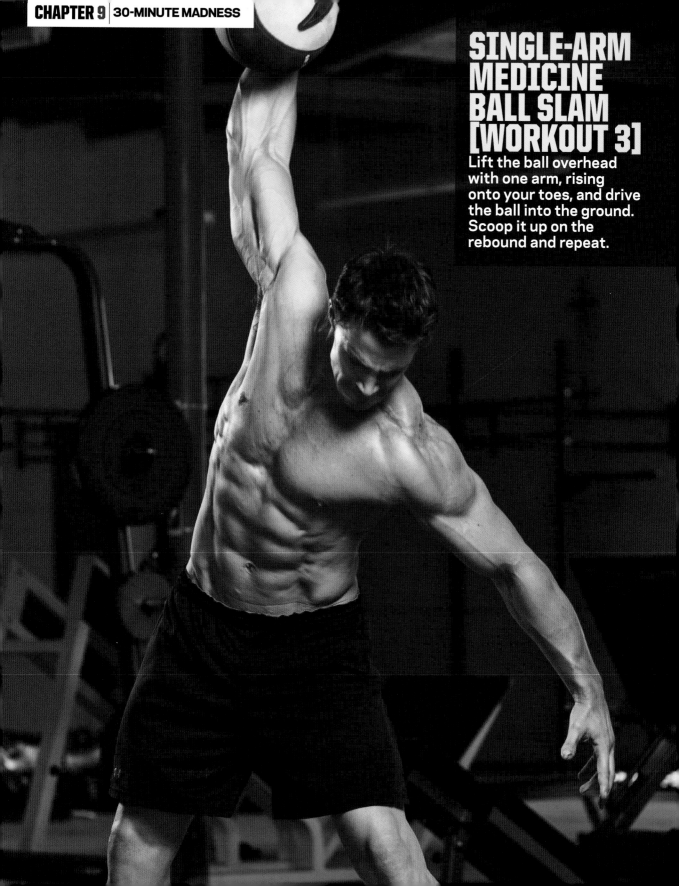

SINGLE-ARM MEDICINE BALL SLAM
[WORKOUT 3]

Lift the ball overhead with one arm, rising onto your toes, and drive the ball into the ground. Scoop it up on the rebound and repeat.

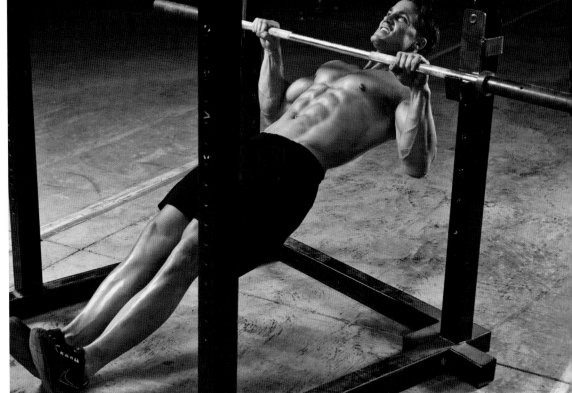

**INVERTED ROW
[WORKOUT 3]**
Set an empty barbell on the lower J-hooks of a power rack (or Smith machine). Keep your abs tight as you pull your chin to the bar.

4

THE UPPER LIMIT
TARGET: CHEST AND BACK

THE IDEA: *This is a basic front-back superset with one major twist—the finishing superset is going to build up areas typically neglected in other programs. Dumbbell scaption hits the stabilizers of your rotator cuff; face pulls hit your rear delts and rhomboids. Complete all the sets in each pair before moving on.*

THE WORKOUT:
1A) Barbell Bench Press: 10,10,8,8
1B) Wide-grip Pullup: 10,10,8,8
2A) DB Incline Press: 3x8
2B) Barbell Bentover Row: 3x8
3A) DB Chest Flye: 3x10
3B) Lat Pulldown: 3x10
4A) DB Scaption: 3x12
4B) Face Pull: 3x12
Trainer: Brian Thompson

5

RUN THE MOUNTAIN
TARGET: TOTAL BODY

THE IDEA: *This challenge is as much mental as it is physical.* After your warmup, you'll perform one rep of each of the following exercises in the first minute, two reps in the second minute, three in the third, and so on until you reach 10 reps. This is "running the mountain." You'll come back down the mountain after 10 reps, hitting nine, eight, seven, and so on until you get back to one rep. You may have tried this before with biceps curls, but with whole-body movements, this is going to hurt a whole lot more.

THE WORKOUT:
Warmup: 10-minute jog or other aerobic activity
DB Squat to Press
DB Romanian Deadlift to Upright Row
Time x Number of reps for each exercise:

0:00 x 1	10:00 x 9
1:00 x 2	11:00 x 8
2:00 x 3	12:00 x 7
3:00 x 4	13:00 x 6
4:00 x 5	14:00 x 5
5:00 x 6	15:00 x 4
6:00 x 7	16:00 x 3
7:00 x 8	17:00 x 2
8:00 x 9	18:00 x 1
9:00 x 10	

Trainer: Jay DeMayo

6

OFF AND RUNNING
TARGET: TOTAL BODY

THE IDEA: *Starting the circuit with a sprint before you move* on to weighted exercises will keep your heart rate elevated throughout the entire workout, even during movements that wouldn't elevate your heart rate otherwise. Finish two rounds.

THE WORKOUT:
Sprint: 20 seconds
Overhead Squat: 1x12
Walking Lunge: 1x12 each leg
Pullup: 1x8
Dip: 1x12
DB Getup: 1x6 each side
Trainer: Jim Smith

7

NO WEIGHTS NECESSARY
TARGET: TOTAL BODY

THE IDEA: *All the moves in this workout are either compound (body-weight squats and pullups), explosive (burpees and box jumps), or require total-body tension (plank). We'll ease you in and out of this one; the meat of the program actually takes only 15 minutes, with the warmup and cooldown lasting another 15 minutes. It sounds light. It's not.*

THE WORKOUT:

Warmup: Jog slowly for five minutes on a treadmill or cardio machine of your choice. Complete three rounds of the following exercises without resting at the end of the circuit. After you finish the plank, hit as many reps as possible within one minute for the remaining exercises.

1:00 Plank	
1:00 Burpees	
1:00 Body-weight Squat	
1:00 Pullup	
1:00 Box Jump	

Cool down with two minutes each of:
Kneeling Hip-flexor Stretch
Hamstring Stretch
Pec Stretch
Glute Stretch

Trainer: Clay Burwell

8

THE CRIPPLER
TARGET: LEGS

THE IDEA: *A mix of heavy weight, high reps, and big compound movements. This might be the longest 30 minutes of your life.*

THE WORKOUT:

Back Squat:
Ascending sets of five reps each, starting at 45 pounds, until you can no longer hit five reps or form breaks down. Once you miss five reps, drop down to a weight you can handle for 20 reps and bang them out immediately. Take only as much time between sets as it takes to change plates. *Example:* **Five reps each of 45, 95, 135, 185, 225, 250, 275, 300, 315, 330 (miss); 185x20**

DB Walking Lunge:
Ascending sets of 10 reps on each leg until form breaks down. Take 45–60 seconds between sets. *Example:* **30s, 35s, 40s, 45s, 50s, 55s (fail)**

Stiff-leg Deadlift: 3x15

Lateral Plate Push: 2x20 steps each side
Lay a 10- or 25-pound plate on the floor and walk laterally, pushing the plate across the floor with the outside of your foot. If the surface of your gym floor isn't conducive to this, wrap an elastic band around your lower legs and walk laterally.

Trainer: Harry Selkow

ZOTTMAN CURL
[WORKOUT 10]

Hold two dumbbells at your sides with your palms facing forward. Curl them up to your shoulders (your palms should now be facing you). Rotate your forearms so your palms face away from you, then lower the weights to your sides.

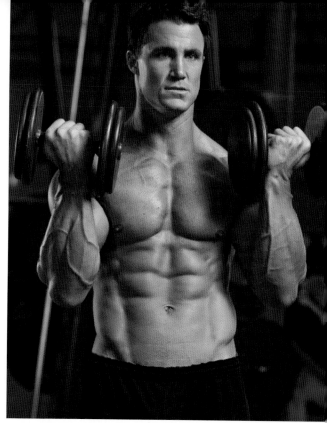

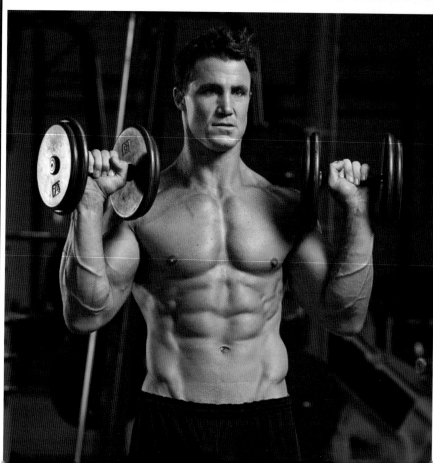

OVERHEAD SQUAT [WORKOUT 6]

Stand in a power rack or squat rack and press a loaded barbell over and slightly behind your head. Contract your abs and keep your elbows locked out as you drop your hips and descend to the floor. Get your thighs at least parallel to the ground, then drive your heels into the floor to return to the starting position.

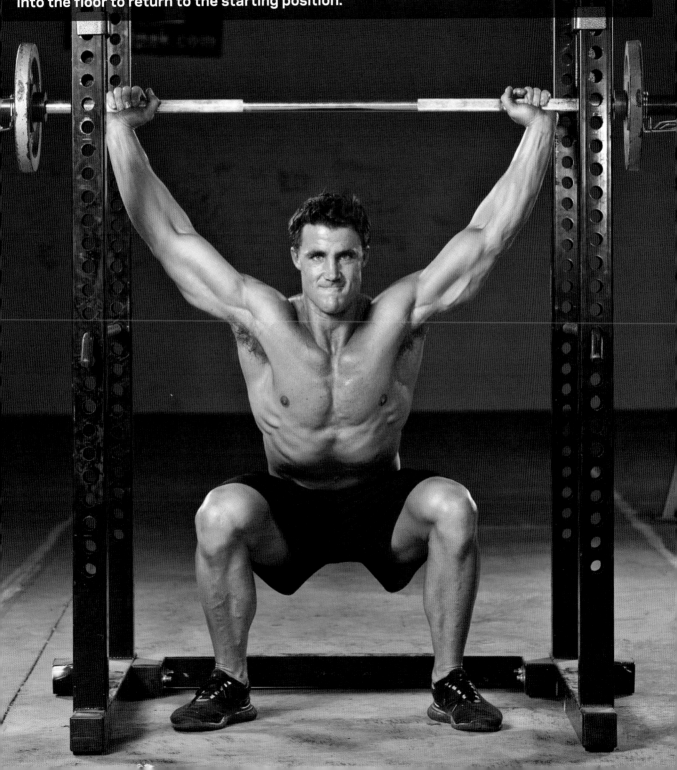

9

DEAD SIMPLE
TARGET: TOTAL BODY

THE IDEA: *The deadlift forces almost every muscle in the body into action. With two different kinds of deadlifts here—plus some heavy upper-body work and a tough finisher for your abs—no muscle is left behind. Don't take any rest between exercises within the pair ("A" and "B"), and rest only 30 seconds at the end of each pair.*

THE WORKOUT:
1) Deadlift: 4x8-10
2A) DB Romanian Deadlift to Upright Row: 3x6-8
2B) Swiss Ball Leg Curl: 3x10
3A) Military Press: 3x10
3B) Chinup: 3x12
4) Ab Wheel Rollout: 3x12

Trainer: Jim Smith

10

THE BIG ARM "SANDWICH"
TARGET: BICEPS AND TRICEPS

THE IDEA: *Start with an isolation exercise, follow it with a compound exercise, and finish with the same isolation exercise (this is the sandwich). The pre-fatigue and long negatives guarantee you'll be walking out of the gym with a swollen set of guns.*

THE WORKOUT:
1A) Zottman Curl: 1x5
Take five seconds on the way down, zero seconds at the bottom, and two seconds on the way up—also known as a 5-0-2 tempo.
1B) Chinup: AMAP
(as many as possible, 4-0-1 tempo)
1C) Zottman Curl: 1x3
(5-0-2 tempo)
Rest 90 seconds and repeat for three total rounds.
2A) Lying Triceps Extension: 1x6 (3-0-2 tempo)
2B) Dip: AMAP (2-0-1 tempo)
2C) Lying Triceps Extension: 1x4 (3-0-2 tempo)
Rest 90 seconds and repeat for three total rounds.

Trainer: Jay DeMayo

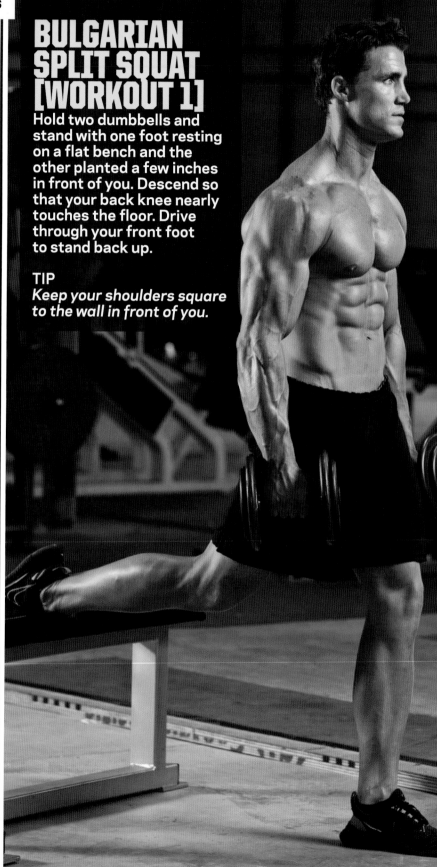

BULGARIAN SPLIT SQUAT [WORKOUT 1]

Hold two dumbbells and stand with one foot resting on a flat bench and the other planted a few inches in front of you. Descend so that your back knee nearly touches the floor. Drive through your front foot to stand back up.

TIP
Keep your shoulders square to the wall in front of you.

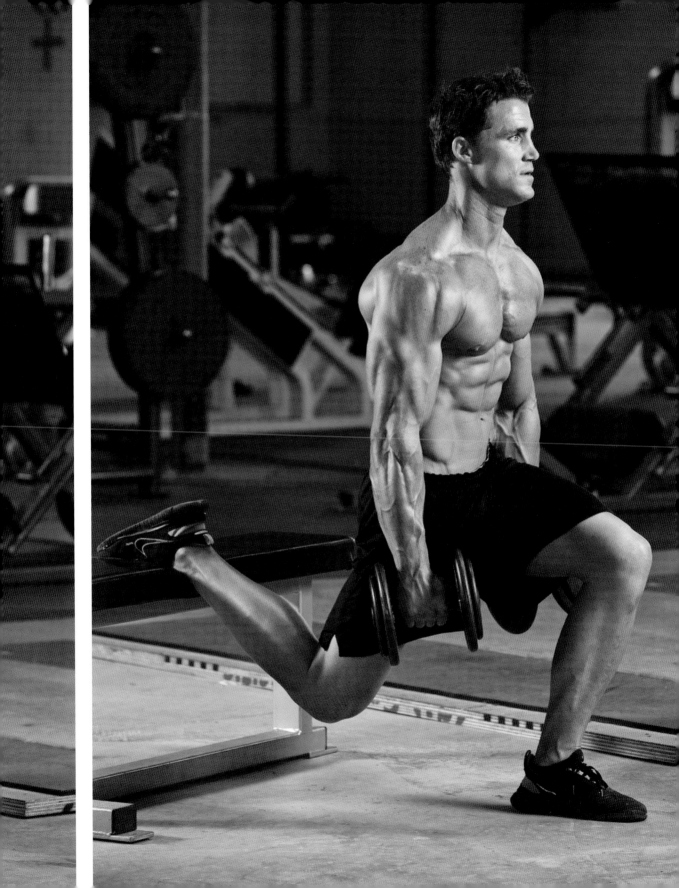

CHAPTER 10

20 30 40 *MINUTES

WORKING LONG HOURS AND HAVING PRECIOUS LITTLE TIME TO TRAIN SUCKS, BUT YOUR WORKOUTS DON'T HAVE TO. STREAMLINE YOUR TRAINING WITH THIS TIME-CONSCIOUS TOTAL-BODY PROGRAM

Once again, it's on. Precious minutes are draining from your schedule, and all the gains you've sweated and bled for all year are at risk of evaporating right before your eyes. That's what happens when reality sets in and work, friends, and family take up the vast majority of your time. But it can all be prevented with a time-efficient full-body routine that leaves no stone—or rock-hard muscle—unturned.

When life makes a regular exercise schedule impossible, it doesn't take long for your body to forget what you've come to expect from it. To avoid this from happening, we've employed trainer Jeff Bell, C.S.C.S., NASM, ACSM, owner of Bell Fitness Co. in New York City, to come up with a plan that will get your body through any busy season unscathed.

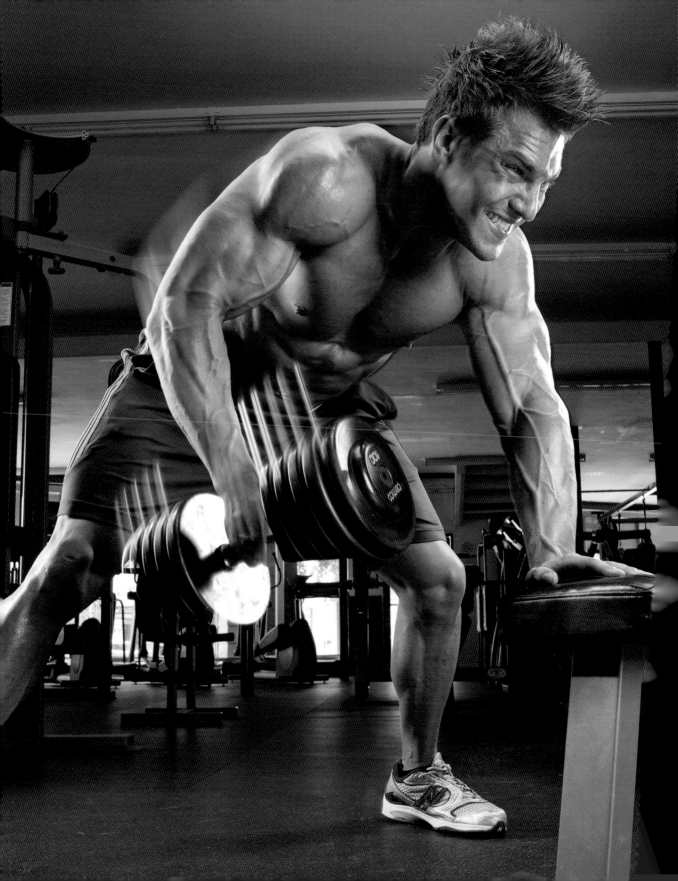

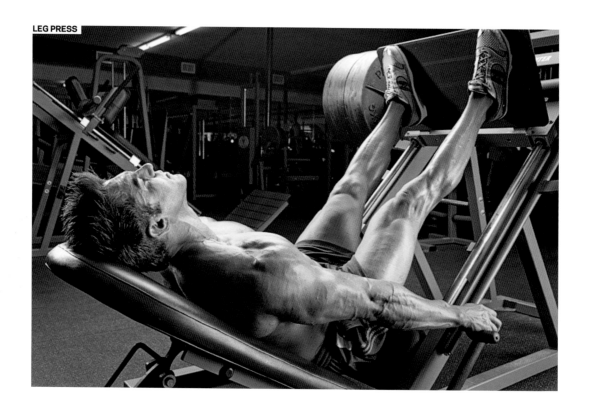

LEG PRESS

THE HARD BASICS

Keeping your hard-earned progress intact in the midst of a hectic schedule doesn't have to be difficult as long as you focus on working the right muscle groups. The idea is to implement a three-days-per-week schedule that relies primarily on heavy, multijoint exercises performed circuit-style to burn more calories and fat. "The smartest choice you can make is a high-intensity full-body plan that stimulates as many muscle fibers as possible," Bell says.

Bell's routine uses some variety of four foundation exercises that target your larger muscle groups (legs, back, and chest) to give you the best possible session in the shortest amount of time. It also includes several unique moves—renegade rows and crucifix shoulder extensions—designed to challenge your body in unfamiliar ways.

"By training your muscles through a greater diversity of angles throughout the week, you'll utilize a greater amount of muscle fibers, which will burn extra calories in the process," Bell says. "You'll also train every possible muscle group at least once a week, if not several times, so they're reminded to stay as strong as possible until you can return to your usual routine."

TIME MANAGEMENT

The primary goal of this workout is to keep your muscles powerful and pumped by taking advantage of the principle of muscle confusion. If you find a few extra minutes to spare on certain days, however, this routine is easily adjustable, with room for up to six more movements and even better results.

The basic template is a full-body routine you'll perform three times a week. If you have 20 minutes to work with, you'll hit four main exercises as a circuit, resting 15–60 seconds between exercises. Working your way through all four moves is one round. Three rounds is the gold standard for a 20-minute session, but if you're feeling particularly energetic, go for four.

With 30 minutes of workout time, add the "bonus" exercise to the template, making each round consist of five moves. For 40 minutes, add the sixth "bonus" move, keeping the circuit-style performance of the rounds the same.

Regardless of how many minutes you're able to exercise each day, Bell recommends taking one day off between sessions. No matter how hard you push your muscles, you'll still need a full 48 hours of recovery to give them enough time to rest and rebuild between your workouts.

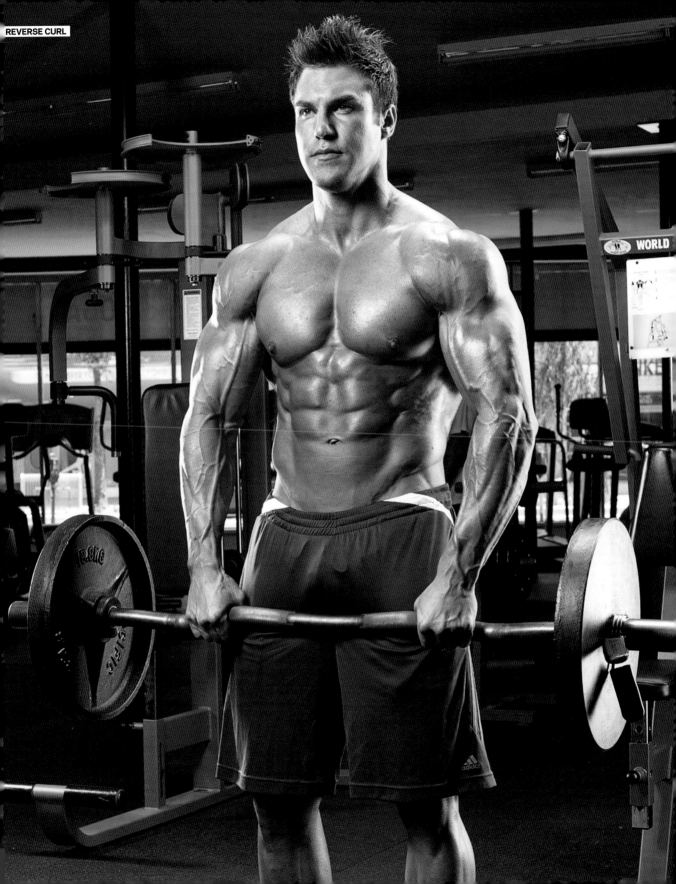

PULLUP

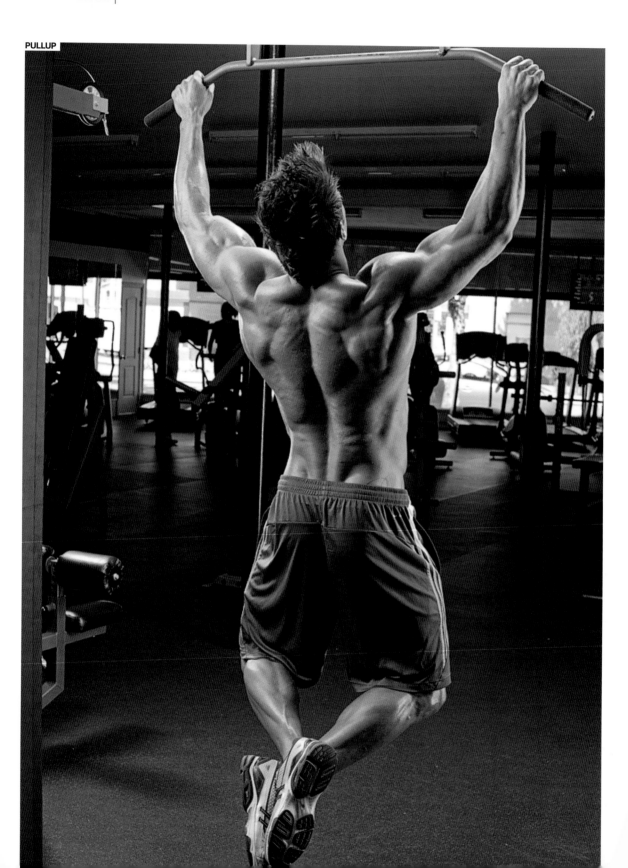

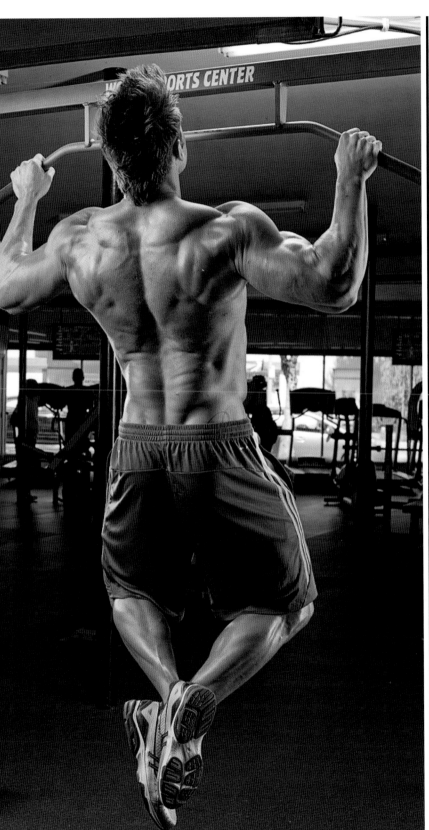

YOUR MONTH-LONG PLAN

EXERCISE	REPS
MONDAY	
Alternating Heavy Dumbbell Chest Press	8-10
Pullup	6-12
Heavy Dumbbell Swing	8-12
Leg Press	8-12
If you have 30 minutes, add…	
Reverse Curl	8-12
If you have 40 minutes, add…	
EZ-bar Lying Triceps Extension	12-15
TUESDAY	Rest
WEDNESDAY	
Back Squat	6-8
Machine Incline Press	8-12
Heavy One-arm Bentover Row	8-12 each side
Hanging Leg Raise	12-15
If you have 30 minutes, add…	
Crucifix Shoulder Extension	8-12
If you have 40 minutes, add…	
Incline Hammer Curl	8-12
THURSDAY	Rest
FRIDAY	
Dumbbell Front Squat	12-15
Parallel-bar Dip	8-15
Renegade Row	8-12
Cable Overhead Triceps Extension	8-12
If you have 30 minutes, add…	
Close-grip Chin	6-12
If you have 40 minutes, add…	
Box Jump	8-10
SATURDAY/SUNDAY	Rest

THE FREQUENCY
MONDAY, WEDNESDAY, FRIDAY

Week 1
Rest 60 seconds between exercises/ circuits; do two rounds

Week 2
Rest 45 seconds between exercises/ circuits; do two rounds

Week 3
Rest 30 seconds between exercises/ circuits; do two to three rounds

Week 4
Rest 15-20 seconds between exercises/ circuits; do three to four rounds

MONDAY - 20 MINUTES
ALTERNATING HEAVY DUMBBELL CHEST PRESS
START: Lie faceup on the floor with your knees bent and your feet flat on the floor. Have a training partner hand you a pair of heavy dumbbells so your arms remain extended, weights directly above your chest.
EXECUTION: Keeping your left arm straight, slowly lower the weight in your right hand until your upper arm touches the floor. Press the dumbbell back up, then repeat with your left arm while keeping your right arm straight. Alternate for reps.

PULLUP
START: Grasp an overhead bar using an overhand grip with your hands slightly wider than shoulder width. Hang from the bar, keeping your arms straight and your elbows unlocked.
EXECUTION: Slowly pull yourself up until your chin passes the bar, then lower yourself back down until your arms are straight.
10-SECOND TIP
If you need to cheat by "kipping" your legs on the last few reps, that's OK.

HEAVY DUMBBELL SWING
START: With your feet wider than shoulder width, squat down and grasp one end of a heavy dumbbell with both hands. Hold the weight between your legs.
EXECUTION: Quickly push yourself into a standing position as you shift your hips forward, and swing the dumbbell up and in front of you to approximately shoulder level. Reverse the move until the weight's once again between your legs.
10-SECOND TIP
Let the dumbbell swing all the way between your legs so you feel the pull in your hamstrings, then extend your hips and explode back up.

LEG PRESS
START: Sit in a leg-press machine with your back and glutes flat against the seat and your feet hip-width apart on the platform.
EXECUTION: Press the weight up until your legs are straight, knees unlocked. Release the safeties and slowly lower the platform until your knees form 90-degree angles.

BONUS MOVES
30-MINUTE MOVE
REVERSE CURL
START: Grasp an EZ-bar or a barbell with an overhand, shoulder-width grip. Your arms should hang straight down so the bar rests in front of your thighs.
EXECUTION: Keeping your back straight and your elbows tucked into your sides, slowly curl the bar up in a semicircular motion until the top of your forearms touch your biceps.

40-MINUTE MOVE
EZ-BAR LYING TRICEPS EXTENSION
START: Lie faceup on a bench holding a loaded EZ-bar with both hands. Extend your arms above your shoulders, perpendicular to the floor, with your palms facing your feet.
EXECUTION: Keeping your upper arms stationary, slowly bend your elbows and lower the bar to your forehead. Straighten your arms to return to the start position.

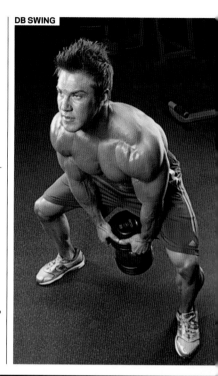

DB SWING

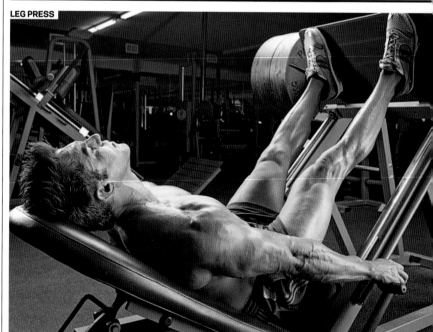

LEG PRESS

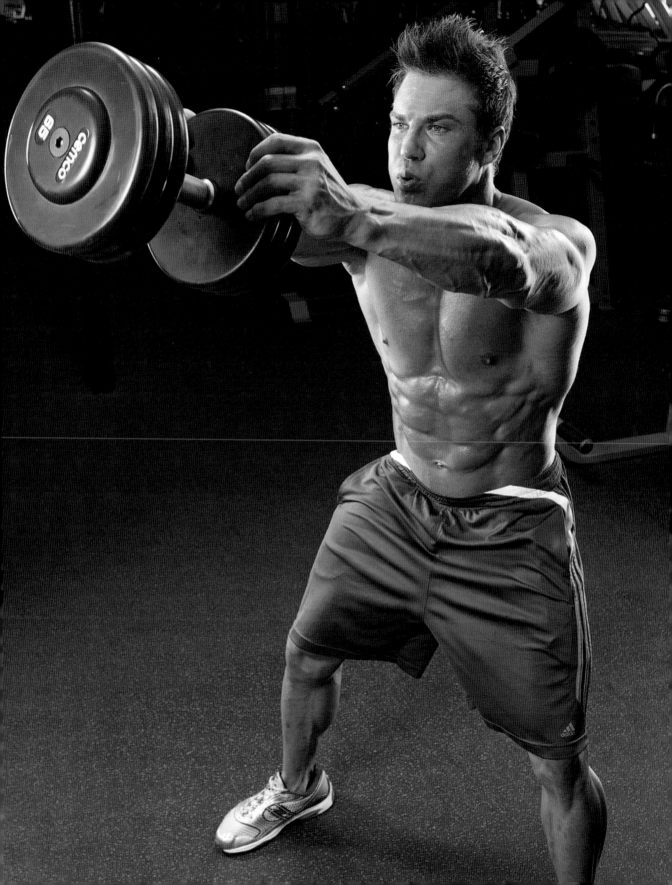

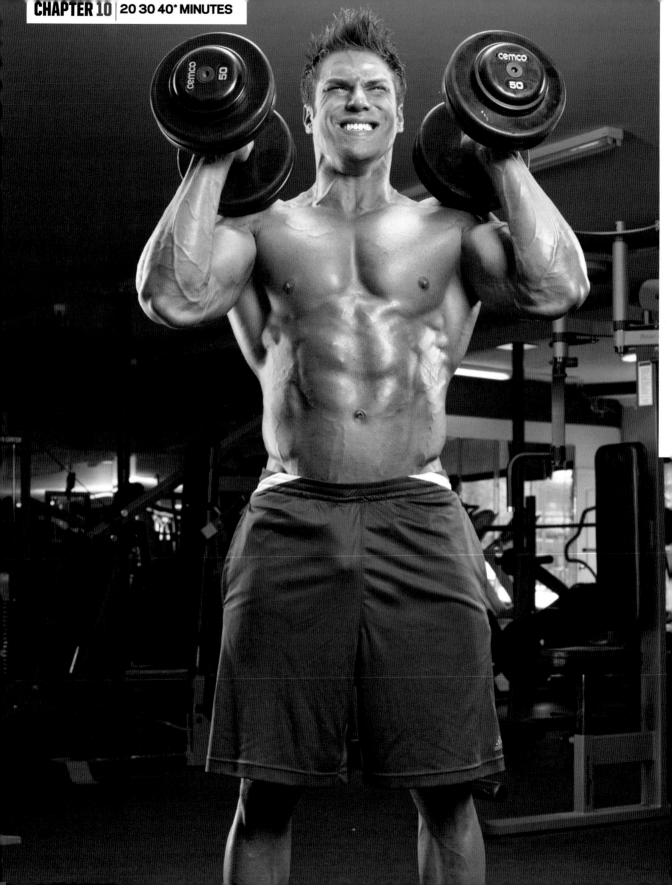

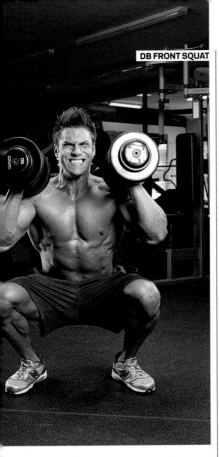

DB FRONT SQUAT

EXECUTION: Press the handles forward until your arms are straight, elbows unlocked, then slowly lower the weight back to the start position.

HANGING LEG RAISE
START: Hang from an overhead bar with your hands wider than shoulder-width apart. Your legs should hang straight underneath you, with your knees slightly bent and your feet pointing down.
EXECUTION: Tilt your pelvis up and slowly raise your legs until they're parallel to the floor, then return to the start. Avoid using momentum; control each rep.

BONUS MOVES
30-MINUTE MOVE
CRUCIFIX SHOULDER EXTENSION
START: Standing at a cable crossover station, remove the handles from the low-pulley cables and grasp the plastic balls with your opposite hands so your arms are crossed in front of you. Bend your elbows 90 degrees and raise them so your fists are in line with your face, with your hands approximately a foot apart.
EXECUTION: Externally rotate your shoulders as you extend your arms overhead. Envision raising your arms as if to throw a softball overhead. Rotate and lower your arms back to the start position.

40-MINUTE MOVE
INCLINE HAMMER CURL
START: Set an adjustable incline bench to 20–30 degrees, then lie faceup on it with a dumbbell in each hand. Your arms should hang down slightly behind your torso.
EXECUTION: Curl the weights to the front of your shoulders, then lower.

FRIDAY - 20 MINUTES
DUMBBELL FRONT SQUAT
START: Hold heavy dumbbells at shoulder level, with your palms facing in and your elbows pointed down. Stand with your feet shoulder-width apart.
EXECUTION: With your back straight and your eyes forward, slowly squat down until your thighs are nearly parallel to the floor, then return to standing.
10-SECOND TIP
Keep your head and chest up, especially on your last few reps. Dumbbell front squats tend to pull you forward, so fight gravity and maintain your upright position.

DIP
START: Grasp the parallel dip bars with your palms facing in. Extend your arms, keeping your elbows unlocked and your knuckles pointing straight down.
execution: Keeping your arms close to your body, bend your elbows and slowly descend until your upper arms are parallel to the floor. Push yourself back up until your arms are straight, elbows unlocked.

RENEGADE ROW
START: Grasp a dumbbell in each hand and get into pushup position with your hands directly below your shoulders and your feet about shoulder-width apart.
EXECUTION: Balancing yourself on one weight, slowly raise the opposite dumbbell to your side. Lower it back to the floor, then switch arms.

CABLE OVERHEAD TRICEPS EXTENSION
START: Attach a rope handle to a high-pulley cable. Grasp each end, then turn around so you face away from the machine. Extend your arms overhead with your palms close together and facing each other, and lean slightly forward. Stand with your feet staggered and your knees slightly bent.
EXECUTION: Keeping your upper arms next to your head, bend your elbows and lower your hands as far behind you as possible. Straighten your arms to return to the start position.

BONUS MOVES
30-MINUTE MOVE
CLOSE-GRIP CHIN
START: Grasp an overhead bar or close-grip handle with an underhand or neutral grip. Your hands should be six to eight inches apart. Hang from the bar with your arms straight and your elbows unlocked.
EXECUTION: Slowly pull yourself up until your chin passes the bar, then lower yourself back down until your arms are straight.

40-MINUTE MOVE
BOX JUMP
START: Set up a stable platform such as a box or bench that's 18–24 inches high, then stand in front of it with your feet hip-width apart, arms bent, and fists facing forward.
EXECUTION: Bend your knees and bring your arms behind you, then swing your arms forward to gain momentum as you jump onto the box. Try to land softly. Step off the box—don't jump off—and quickly assume the start position.

WEDNESDAY - 20 MINUTES
BACK SQUAT
START: With your hands slightly wider than shoulder width, grasp a barbell with an overhand grip and rest it across your shoulders. Lift the bar off the rack and step back.
EXECUTION: With your back straight and your feet shoulder-width apart, descend until your thighs are almost parallel to the floor, then slowly press back up to standing.

HEAVY ONE-ARM BENTOVER ROW
START: Stand alongside a flat bench with a heavy dumbbell in your left hand. Place your right hand on the bench for support, then step your feet backward until your back is almost parallel to the floor. Your left arm should hang straight down with your palm facing in.
EXECUTION: Holding this position, slowly pull the weight close to your body until it reaches your side. Lower the dumbbell and repeat for reps, then switch sides.

MACHINE INCLINE PRESS
START: Sit in the machine with your feet flat on the floor, and your head, back and glutes flat against the seat. Grasp the handles in front of you with an overhand grip.

CHAPTER 11

FIND THE
PERFECT
WORKOUT

LOOKING FOR WORKOUTS TO TARGET SPECIFIC MUSCLE GROUPS? YOU'VE COME TO THE RIGHT PLACE. MULTIPLE ROUTINES FOR EVERY BODY PART—68 IN ALL—COVERING EVERY GOAL FROM MASS-GAINING TO STRENGTH-BUILDING TO BRINGING UP WEAK AREAS.

High-level trainers agree on very little outside of the fact that there's no such thing as a one-size-fits-all routine. If we all had the same training goals and body types, we'd all look like a young Arnold. But we have different wants and needs; some of us want size, others want a bigger squat or a wider back, and there are those who need to train at home, which led us to offer you a complete menu of workouts for every major body part that covers all desirable objectives and circumstances. So feel free to pick and choose from the wide array of routines contained in the following pages. Because there's no reason you can't create the program you need for the body you want.

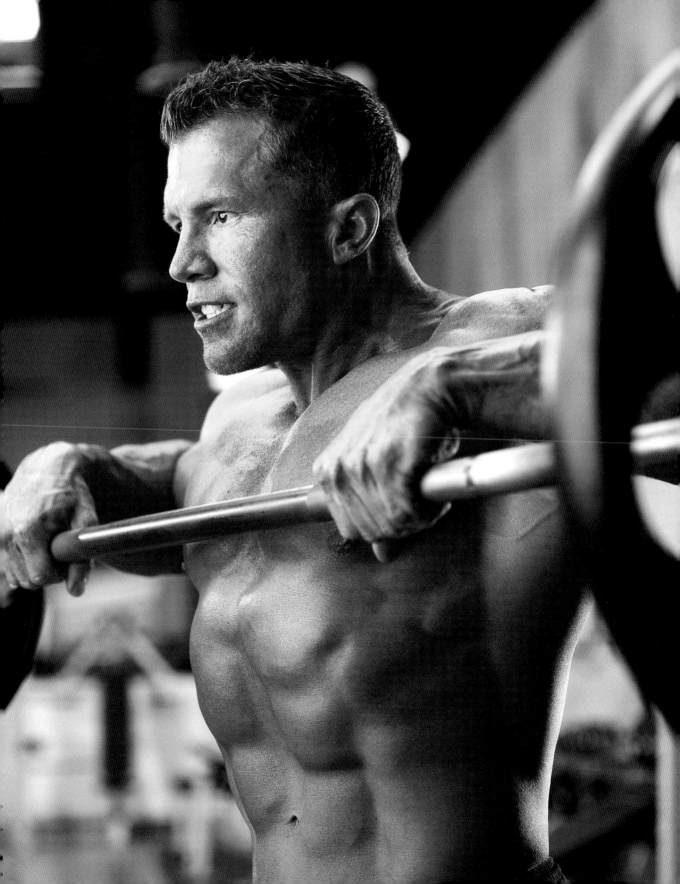

ROUTINE RUNDOWN

Here's a brief description of the different categories of workouts you'll find on the following pages:

MASS-BUILDING
Exercise selection, volume, and rep ranges specifically intended for packing on mass

BEGINNER'S
Basic, introductory routines for trainees with fewer than six months of training under their belts

AT-HOME
Workouts that require nothing more than dumbbells, an adjustable bench, and a set of elastic bands—a common home-gym setup

15-MINUTE
Brief but intense sessions ideally suited for those short on time but seeking big results (for abs, it's a 10-minute workout)

"PRIORITY"
Routines designed to bring up common lagging areas, such as the biceps "peak" and the lower abs, or emphasize particular training aspects like full range of motion for legs

STRENGTH/POWER
Big exercises, low reps, and generous rest periods to help boost explosiveness and one-rep-max strength

PREHAB/REHAB
Workouts intended to help you avoid common injuries (prehab) or strengthen areas that have been injured (rehab)

CIRCUIT
Fast-paced routines that maximize intensity for a particular muscle group by attacking it with multiple exercises performed consecutively without rest

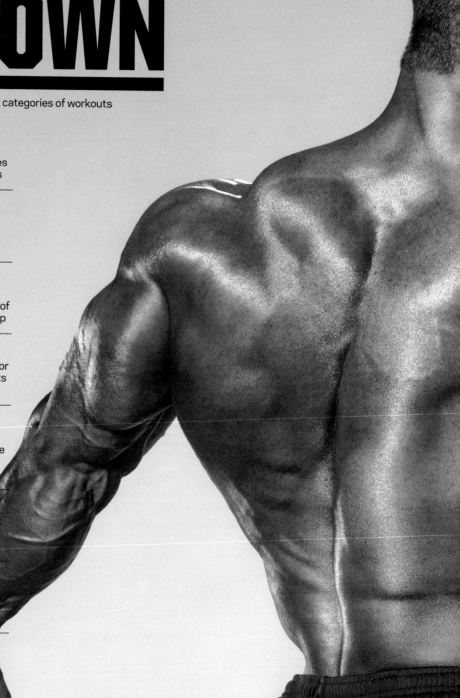

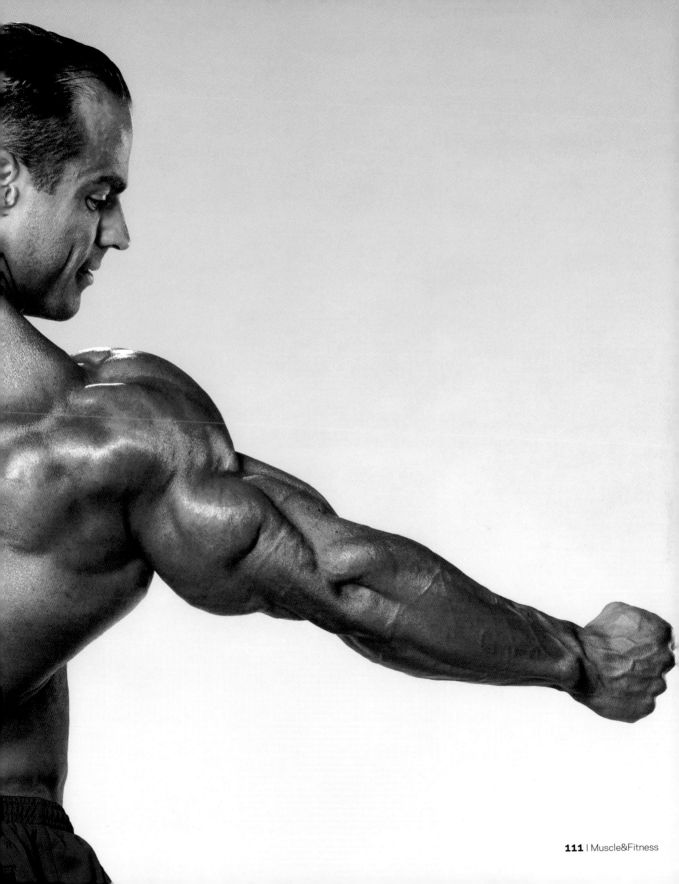

CHEST

MASS-BUILDING WORKOUT IN FOCUS

Packing on size requires two major training factors: high volume and moderate rep ranges. This routine satisfies both with 16 total sets, five of them coming from the old standby barbell bench press and another five from cable crossovers as a finishing move that isolates the pecs to increase muscle pump and maximize hypertrophy. The ideal rep range for mass is 8–12, thus every set in this routine falls in that range. The workout also includes incline and decline presses to hit the chest from all angles and exhaust every last muscle fiber, another key to growth.

MASS-BUILDING

EXERCISE	SETS	REPS
Bench Press	5	8
Dumbbell Incline Press	3	12
Decline Bench Press	3	12
Cable Crossover	5	10

LIFTING LOWDOWN

If there's one body part in particular that's prone to a training rut, it's chest. Switch things up constantly. Alternate between doing flat and incline presses first in your workout. Don't always go heavy on presses and light on flyes; reverse the order sometimes.

DECLINE BENCH PRESS

After touching the bar to your lower pecs, press it straight up (perpendicular to the floor) instead of in a backward arc like you do with flat-bench presses.

WEIGHTED DIP

On chest day, lean forward when dipping to target the pecs; keeping your body upright puts more emphasis on the triceps.

TIP: SPLIT DECISION

Chest pairs well with shoulders and triceps in a push-pull legs split or with back in an upper body–lower body split.

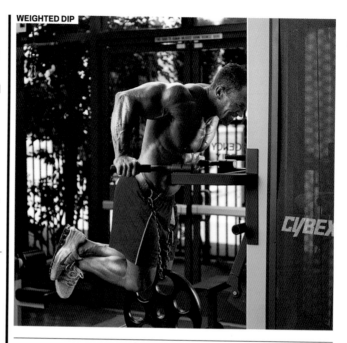

WEIGHTED DIP

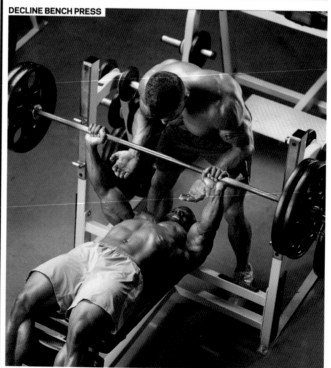

DECLINE BENCH PRESS

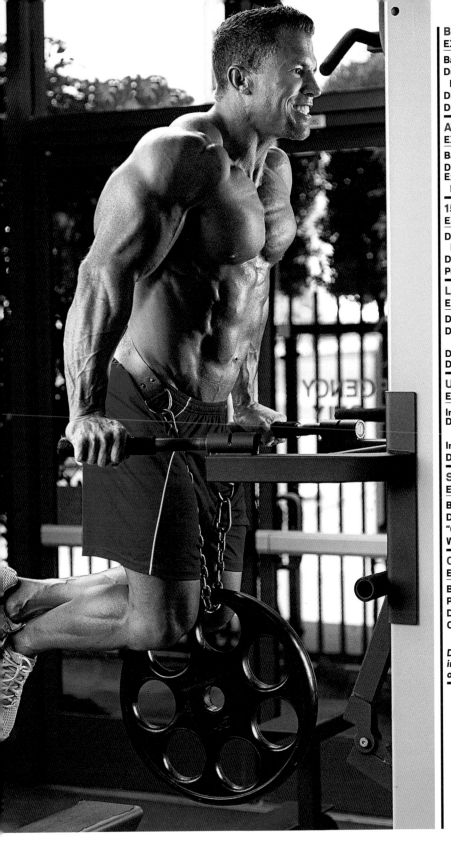

BEGINNER'S

EXERCISE	SETS	REPS
Barbell Pushup	3	10
Dumbbell Bench Press	3	10
Dip	3	10
Dumbbell Flye	3	10

AT-HOME

EXERCISE	SETS	REPS
Banded Pushup	3	20
Dumbbell Floor Press	3	12
Exercise-ball Dumbbell Flye	3	12

15-MINUTE

EXERCISE	SETS	REPS
Dumbbell Bench Press	3	15
Decline Pushup	3	15
Pec-deck Flye	3	20

LOWER-CHEST PRIORITY

EXERCISE	SETS	REPS
Decline Bench Press	3	12
Decline Dumbbell Press	3	12
Decline Flye	3	15
Dip	3	To failure

UPPER-CHEST PRIORITY

EXERCISE	SETS	REPS
Incline Bench Press	3	12
Dumbbell Incline Press	3	12
Incline Cable Flye	3	15
Decline Pushup	3	12

STRENGTH/POWER

EXERCISE	SETS	REPS
Bench Press	5	5
Dumbbell Floor Press	3	6
"Clap" Pushup	5	5
Weighted Dip	3	To failure

CIRCUIT

EXERCISE	SETS	REPS
Bench Press	4	10
Pushup	4	10
Dip	4	10
One-arm Alternating Dumbbell Press	4	10 each side

Do one set of each movement without resting. Perform the circuit four times, resting one to two minutes between each round.

BACK

UPPER-LATS PRIORITY WORKOUT IN FOCUS

Targeting the upper lats, which lie just below the armpits, creates overall back width and contributes greatly to the much-desired V-taper physique. Wide-grip pullups are the king of back-widening moves, which is why we chose them to kick off the workout. Do as many reps as possible on every set to force your lats to grow. Face pulls also zero in on the upper lats. Simply stand in front of a lat pulldown machine, put one foot up on the seat to stabilize yourself, grasp the rope or bar (the latter with a wide grip) and pull it straight to your forehead in a rowing fashion.

UPPER-LATS PRIORITY

EXERCISE	SETS	REPS
Wide-grip Pullup	3	To failure
Rope Face Pull	3	15
Face Pull	3	15
Wide-grip Seated Cable Row	3	10

LIFTING LOWDOWN

Whichever back exercise you're doing, whether it's a pulldown, row, or pullup, always concentrate on squeezing your shoulder blades together as you pull the weight. This ensures the majority of the stress is placed on your back muscles, not your biceps.

ONE-ARM DUMBBELL ROW

Keep your torso parallel to the floor throughout, even at the top of the rep; don't open your shoulder as you pull the weight up.

CLOSE-GRIP LAT PULLDOWN

Concentrate on your lower lats during this exercise by pointing your elbows straight down, not back.

SPLIT DECISION

Hitting back and biceps together (back first, of course) is your classic pull workout. Back can be paired with most any body part, but avoid it on hardcore leg days.

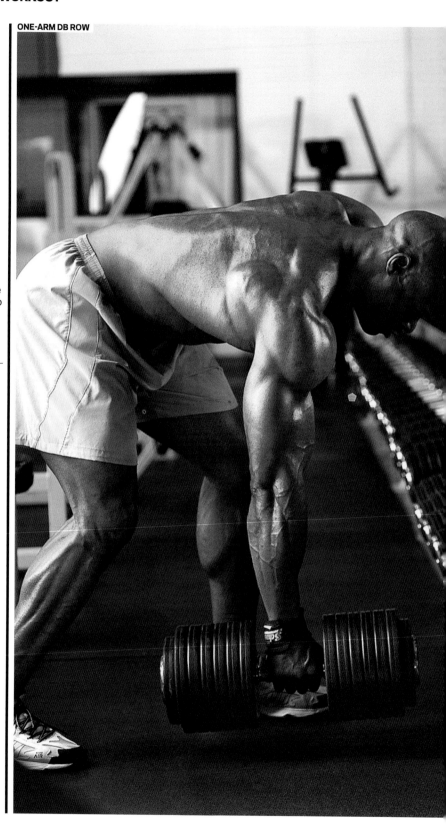

ONE-ARM DB ROW

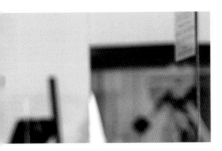

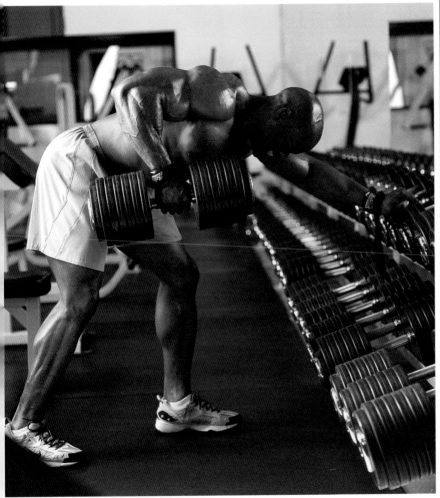

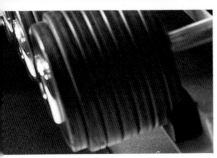

MASS-BUILDING

EXERCISE	SETS	REPS
Pullup	3	To failure
Bentover Row	5	10
One-arm Dumbbell Row	3	10 each side
Lat Pulldown	5	10

BEGINNER'S

EXERCISE	SETS	REPS
Lat Pulldown	3	10
Close-grip Lat Pulldown	3	10
Seated Cable Row	3	10
Standing Low-cable Row	3	10

AT-HOME

EXERCISE	SETS	REPS
Dumbbell Row	5	10
Dumbbell Pullover	5	10
Banded Doorway Face Pull	5	10

15-MINUTE

EXERCISE	SETS	REPS
Lat Pulldown	3	20
Face Pull	3	20
Dumbbell "Kroc" Row	1	To failure

LOWER-LATS PRIORITY

EXERCISE	SETS	REPS
Chin	3	10
T-bar Row	3	10
Bentover Row	3	10
Close-grip Lat Pulldown	3	10

STRENGTH/POWER

EXERCISE	SETS	REPS
Weighted Pullup	3	6
Bentover Row	5	6
Dumbbell Row	5	6
"Dead-stop" Bentover Row*	3	6

*Allow weight to rest on the floor between each rep.

CIRCUIT

EXERCISE	SETS	REPS
Bentover Row	4	10
Underhand Bentover Row	4	10
Inverted Row	4	10
Underhand Inverted Row	4	10

Do one set of each movement without resting. Perform the circuit four times, resting oone to two minutes between each round.

SHOULDERS/ TRAPS

UPRIGHT ROW

DELTS PRIORITY WORKOUT IN FOCUS

Isolating the deltoids from the traps isn't as easy as it may seem. When doing the three raise variations (bentover, lateral, front), don't shrug up as you lift the dumbbells, but lift through the entire range of motion with only your delts. Same goes for seated overhead presses. The Cuban rotation is a novel exercise that's great for isolating the front delts and rotator cuffs. Hold a light barbell directly in front of your shoulders with your elbows bent 90 degrees. Keeping your upper arms stationary, rotate your shoulders to pull the bar toward your forehead.

DELTS PRIORITY

EXERCISE	SETS	REPS
Seated Overhead Press	3	12
Cuban Rotation	3	10
Dumbbell Bentover Lateral Raise	3	10
Dumbbell Lateral Raise	3	10
Dumbbell Front Raise	3	10

UPRIGHT ROW

Focus on keeping your shoulders down (depressed) as you pull the bar up against your body. This will keep maximum tension on the delts.

DUMBBELL OVERHEAD PRESS

Don't lock out your elbows at the top of the rep. Doing so will only increase your risk of injury and take stress off the delts.

LIFTING LOWDOWN

The shoulders are arguably the easiest body part to injure, as these ball-and-socket joints are inherently unstable. Because of this, ample rest days between hard delt workouts are crucial. If you work shoulders on Monday, don't bench-press on Tuesday.

SPLIT DECISION

Delts can be trained with virtually any body part. Chest and back workouts both directly involve the shoulders, as do Olympic moves such as cleans and snatches.

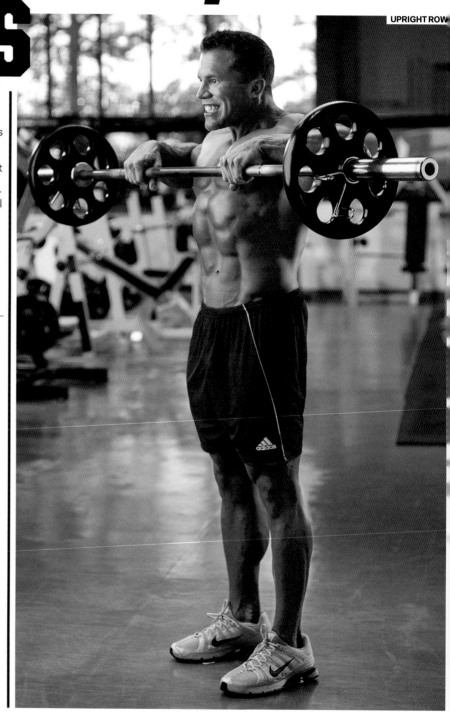

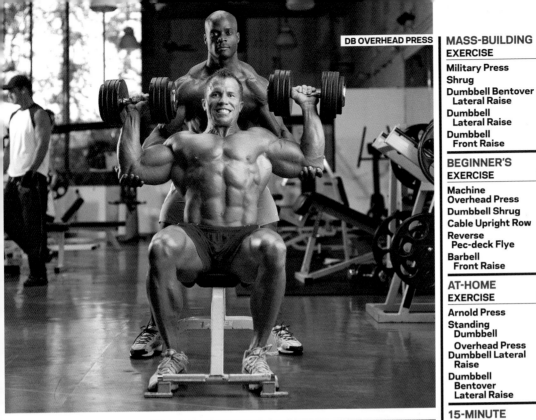

DB OVERHEAD PRESS

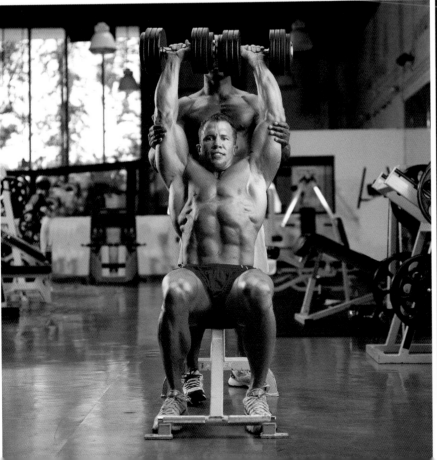

MASS-BUILDING

EXERCISE	SETS	REPS
Military Press	3	12
Shrug	3	15
Dumbbell Bentover Lateral Raise	3	10
Dumbbell Lateral Raise	3	10
Dumbbell Front Raise	3	10

BEGINNER'S

EXERCISE	SETS	REPS
Machine Overhead Press	3	10
Dumbbell Shrug	3	10
Cable Upright Row	3	10
Reverse Pec-deck Flye	3	10
Barbell Front Raise	3	10

AT-HOME

EXERCISE	SETS	REPS
Arnold Press	3	12
Standing Dumbbell Overhead Press	3	12
Dumbbell Lateral Raise	3	10
Dumbbell Bentover Lateral Raise	3	10

15-MINUTE

EXERCISE	SETS	REPS
Barbell Clean and Press	3	8
Shrug	3	15
Upright Row	3	10

TRAPS PRIORITY

EXERCISE	SETS	REPS
Shrug	3	10
Dumbbell Shrug	3	15
One-arm Cable Shrug	3	20 each side

STRENGTH/POWER

EXERCISE	SETS	REPS
Standing Military Press	3	6
Push Press	3	6
Heavy Shrug	5	5
Bentover/Lateral/ Front Raise Superset	3	8

CIRCUIT

EXERCISE	SETS	REPS
Dumbbell Overhead Press	4	12
Dumbbell Upright Row	4	12
Dumbbell Shrug	4	12
Dumbbell Clean	4	12

Do one set of each movement without resting. Perform the circuit four times, resting one to two minutes between each round.

QUADS/GLUTES

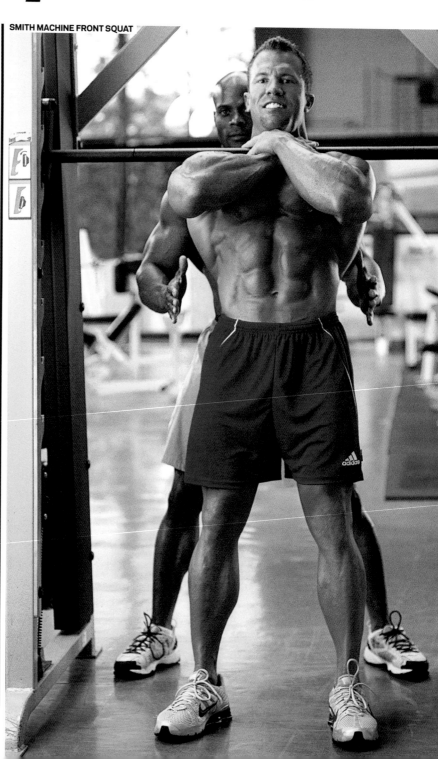

SMITH MACHINE FRONT SQUAT

KNEE-STABILITY PRIORITY WORKOUT IN FOCUS

Possessing stability in the knees is paramount for any athlete (competitive and recreational alike) and serious lifter, both to maximize lower-body strength for enhanced performance and to minimize injury risk. One major key to increasing knee stability is strengthening the vastus medialis muscle (the "teardrop" of the quads), which helps hold the knee joint together.

Shortening the range of motion on box squats and step-ups, and going heavy does just that. When doing box squats, using a taller box than normal will limit how far you can come down; likewise, on step-ups a lower box or step will decrease range of motion.

KNEE-STABILITY PRIORITY

EXERCISE	SETS	REPS
Heavy High-Box Squat[1]	4	8
Heavy Low Step-up[1]	3	10
One-leg Squat	3	8 each side
Half-leg Press[2]	3	10

[1] Use a taller box and lower step, respectively, to decrease range of motion.
[2] Lower the weight only half as far as you normally do on leg presses.

HACK SQUAT

Keeping your feet close together on the platform will target the outer quads; a wider stance hits the inner quads more.

SMITH MACHINE FRONT SQUAT

When setting up, position your feet directly beneath you instead of out in front; this will place more tension on the quads rather than the glutes.

LIFTING LOWDOWN

Shying away from the big lifts (squats, lunges, step-ups) won't help you get bigger legs. Leg extensions have their place, but not as a foundational exercise.

SPLIT DECISION

Training quads on their own is a sufficiently taxing workout, so there's no need to do much else. It makes sense, however, to train hamstrings and calves along with them.

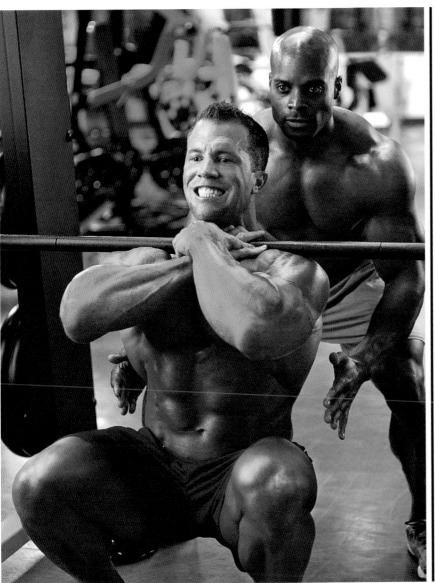

MASS-BUILDING

EXERCISE	SETS	REPS
Smith Machine Front Squat	5	10
Barbell Lunge	3	10
Barbell Reverse Lunge	3	10
One-leg Press	3	10 each side

BEGINNER'S

EXERCISE	SETS	REPS
Body-weight Squat	5	10
Leg Press	3	10
Dumbbell Lunge	3	10

AT-HOME

EXERCISE	SETS	REPS
Dumbbell Front Squat	3	15
Dumbbell Lunge	3	10
Dumbbell Reverse Lunge	3	10
Dumbbell Step-up	3	10

15-MINUTE

EXERCISE	SETS	REPS
Power Squat	3	12
Hack Squat	3	12
Leg Press	3	20

FULL-RANGE-OF-MOTION PRIORITY

EXERCISE	SETS	REPS
Back Squat	3	10
One-leg Squat[1]	3	8 each side
High Step-up[2]	3	10
Reverse Lunge	3	10

1 Front foot elevated

2 Use a taller box or step to increase the range of motion.

STRENGTH/POWER

EXERCISE	SETS	REPS
Box Jump	5	5
Back Squat	5	5
Overhead Squat	3	10
Walking Dumbbell Lunge	3	8

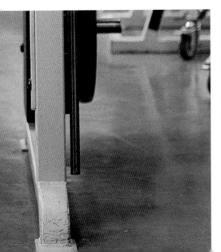

HACK SQUAT

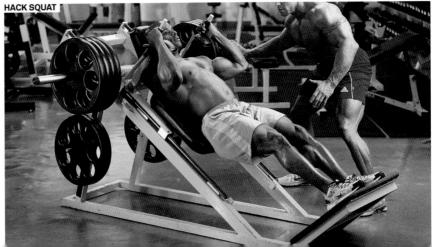

BICEPS

CIRCUIT WORKOUT IN FOCUS

Sometimes a stubborn body part just needs some shock therapy to break through a plateau. You might not think to design a circuit for smaller body parts like biceps, but the high intensity of such a workout just might give your arms the massive pump they need to start growing again. In this circuit, the first three exercises consist of a hammer-curl dropset where you strip enough weight after each set so you can complete 10 reps without resting. After that, grasp a weight plate in front of you with your elbows at your sides and bent 90 degrees for half a minute. This is going to hurt.

CIRCUIT

EXERCISE	SETS	REPS
Hammer Curl	4	10
Hammer Curl (drop 5-10 pounds)	4	10
Hammer Curl (drop 5-10 pounds)	4	10
Static 90-degree Plate Hold	4	30 sec.

Do one set of each movement without resting. Perform the circuit four times, resting one to two minutes between each round.

CLOSE-GRIP BARBELL CURL

Taking a narrow grip on barbell curls—inside shoulder width—targets the long head of the biceps (the "peak").

DUMBBELL PREACHER CURL

As you reach the top of the curl, turn your pinky fingers out (supination) and squeeze your biceps to maximize the contraction.

SPLIT DECISION

Train biceps after back on your "pull" days, or work them with triceps on a dedicated arm day if you're trying to bring up a weak pair of guns.

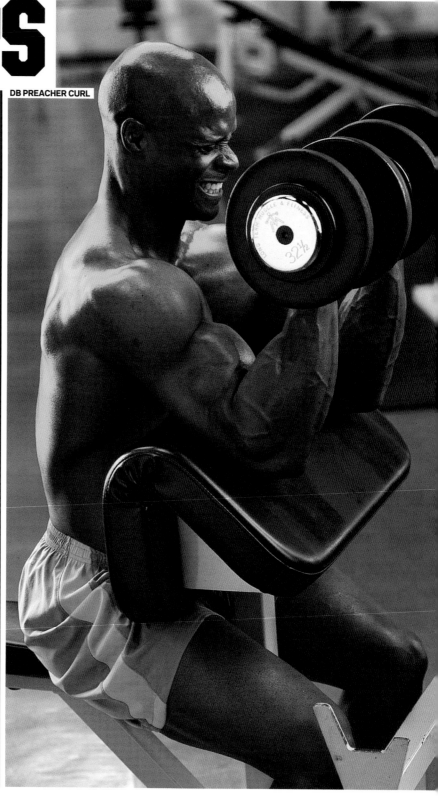

DB PREACHER CURL

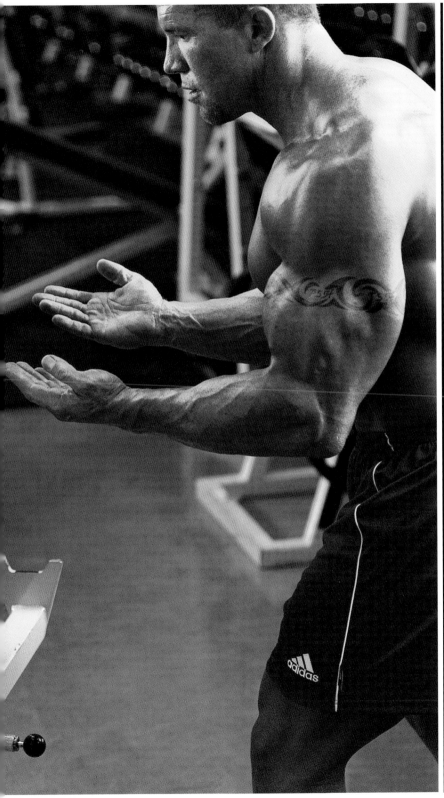

LIFTING LOWDOWN

There's really only one basic movement you can do for biceps: the curl. But don't let that limit your exercise variety. You can do dozens of curling variations to hit the muscles from different angles and spur new growth.

MASS-BUILDING

EXERCISE	SETS	REPS
Barbell Curl	4	10
Hammer Curl	4	10
Dumbbell Incline Curl	4	10
Preacher Curl	4	10

BEGINNER'S

EXERCISE	SETS	REPS
EZ-bar Curl	3	10
Standing Dumbbell Curl	3	10
Reverse Curl	3	10

AT-HOME

EXERCISE	SETS	REPS
Zottman Curl	4	10
Concentration Curl	4	10
Banded Curl	3	To failure

15-MINUTE

EXERCISE	SETS	REPS
Cable Curl	4	10
Reverse Cable Curl	4	10
Cable Preacher Curl	4	10

BICEPS LONG-HEAD PRIORITY

EXERCISE	SETS	REPS
Close-grip Chinup	3	To failure
Close-grip Barbell Curl	3	10
Hammer Curl	3	12
Cable Rope Curl	3	15

BICEPS SHORT-HEAD PRIORITY

EXERCISE	SETS	REPS
Preacher Curl	3	10
Dumbbell Preacher Curl	3	10
Dumbbell Incline Curl	3	10
Wide-grip Barbell Curl	3	10

STRENGTH/POWER

EXERCISE	SETS	REPS
Weighted Chinup	3	To failure
Barbell Curl	4	6
Hammer Curl	4	6
Cable Curl	4	6

TRICEPS

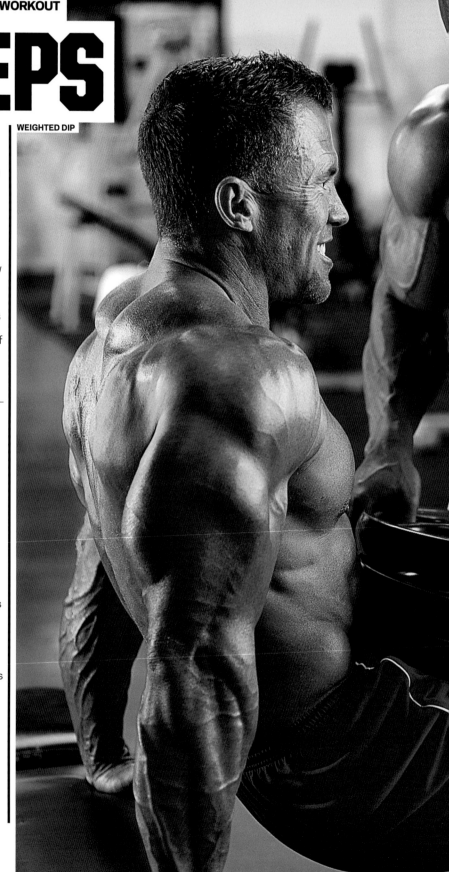

WEIGHTED DIP

STRENGTH/POWER WORKOUT IN FOCUS

Boosting strength and power in the triceps produces two desirable benefits: 1) it increases arm size by overloading the tri's with heavy weights, and 2) it drastically improves your performance in multijoint pressing exercises, namely the bench press and military press. In this workout, close-grip bench presses and weighted dips—two compound triceps moves—allow you to load up on weight for big strength gains. The JM press, a great exercise for increasing bench-press lockout strength, is basically a close-grip bench press (hands 12–18 inches apart) in which the bar is lowered to about the collarbones instead of the pecs with the elbows pointed forward rather than out to the sides.

STRENGTH/POWER

EXERCISE	SETS	REPS
Close-grip Bench Press	5	5
JM Press	3	8
Weighted Dip	3	10
Dumbbell Lying Triceps Extension	3	8

WEIGHTED BENCH DIP

Weighted bench dips make for a great dropset, where your partner takes one weight plate off your lap each time you reach failure.

SEATED DUMBBELL OVERHEAD TRICEPS EXTENSION

A low-back seat is ideal for this exercise, as it provides lower-back support and won't get in the way as you lower the dumbbell behind your head.

LIFTING LOWDOWN

Building the biggest triceps possible means keeping your elbows in, locking them out at the top of each rep and squeezing them for the full contraction, regardless of what exercise you're doing.

SPLIT DECISION

On "push" days, pair triceps with chest and shoulders, or group them with biceps on arm days. Supersetting biceps and triceps is great for building big arms.

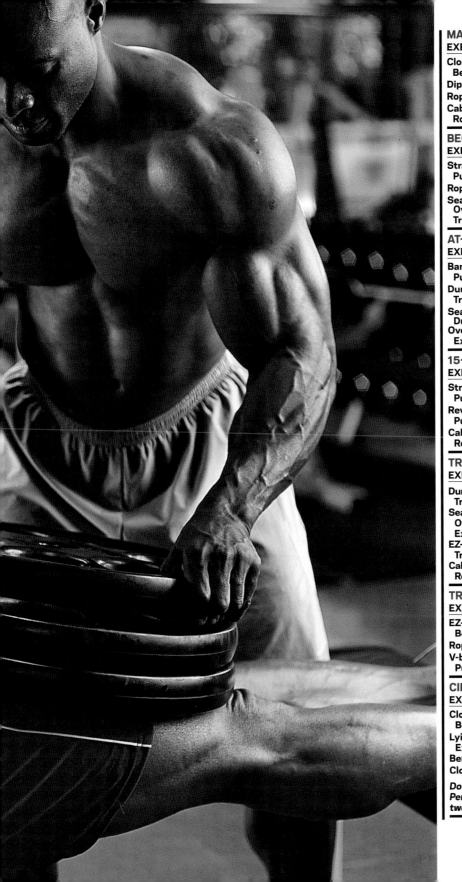

MASS-BUILDING

EXERCISE	SETS	REPS
Close-grip Bench Press	4	10
Dip	4	To failure
Rope Pushdown	4	10
Cable Overhead Rope Extension	4	10

BEGINNER'S

EXERCISE	SETS	REPS
Straight-bar Pushdown	3	10
Rope Pushdown	3	10
Seated Dumbbell Overhead Triceps Extension	3	10

AT-HOME

EXERCISE	SETS	REPS
Banded Close-grip Pushup	3	10
Dumbbell Lying Triceps Extension	3	15
Seated One-arm Dumbbell Overhead Triceps Extension	3	12 each side

15-MINUTE

EXERCISE	SETS	REPS
Straight-bar Pushdown	4	12
Reverse-grip Pushdown	4	12
Cable Overhead Rope Extension	4	12

TRICEPS LONG-HEAD PRIORITY

EXERCISE	SETS	REPS
Dumbbell Lying Triceps Extension	3	12
Seated Dumbbell Overhead Triceps Extension	3	12
EZ-bar Lying Triceps Extension	3	12
Cable Overhead Rope Extension	3	12

TRICEPS LATERAL-HEAD PRIORITY

EXERCISE	SETS	REPS
EZ-bar Close-grip Bench Press	3	12
Rope Pushdown	3	15
V-bar Pushdown	3	15

CIRCUIT

EXERCISE	SETS	REPS
Close-grip Bench Press	4	10
Lying Triceps Extension	4	10
Bench Dip	4	10
Close-grip Pushup	4	10

Do one set of each movement without resting. Perform the circuit four times, resting one to two minutes between each round.

ABS

AT-HOME WORKOUT IN FOCUS

Not having enough time is a lousy excuse for not fitting in your abdominal work—the six-pack is the easiest body part to train at home with zero equipment. This workout hits all areas of the midsection (upper abs, lower abs, obliques, and core) with basic yet effective moves. After crunches, raise your feet off the floor, bend your knees 90 degrees, and bring each elbow to the opposite knee for oblique crunches, alternating sides. The static-crunch hold is exactly what it sounds like: an isometric hold in the top position of the crunch.

AT-HOME

EXERCISE	SETS	REPS
Crunch	3	20
Leg-Raised Oblique Crunch	3	20
Static-Crunch Hold	3	20 sec.
Plank	3	20 sec.

DOUBLE CRUNCH

Use a slow to moderate rep speed to isolate the abs. Moving too quickly will hurt your form and involve too many other muscles.

DECLINE RUSSIAN TWIST

Keep your torso somewhere between parallel and perpendicular to the floor to keep constant tension on the abs as you twist.

LIFTING LOWDOWN

The midsection is a complex, oft-misunderstood group of muscles. It needs to be able to flex and twist the torso, but it's also a critical stabilizer when other muscles are working. So train it as such: Do explosive reps, slow reps, isometric holds, high reps, and low reps.

SPLIT DECISION

Abs can be trained almost every day and with any body part. On leg days, however, be sure to do ab work after big lifts like squats, since a fatigued core can hinder performance.

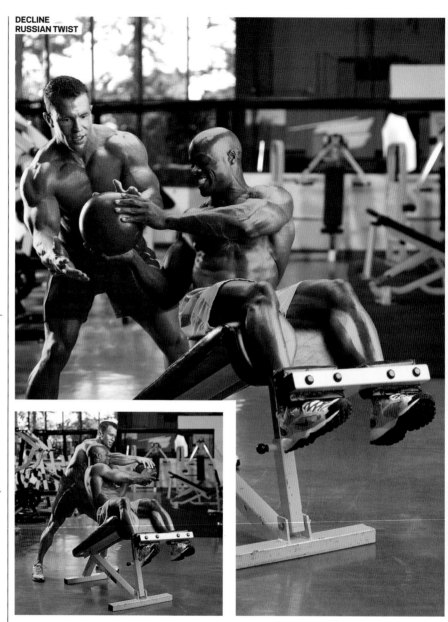

DECLINE RUSSIAN TWIST

BEGINNER'S

EXERCISE	SETS	REPS
Incline Situp	3	10
Crunch	3	10
Plank	3	15 sec.

10-MINUTE

EXERCISE	SETS	REPS
Hanging Leg Raise	3	15
Incline Situp	3	15
Double Crunch	3	15

UPPER ABS/OBLIQUES PRIORITY

EXERCISE	SETS	REPS
Decline Russian Twist	3	10
Machine Crunch	3	15
Standing Cable Crunch	3	15

LOWER-ABS PRIORITY

EXERCISE	SETS	REPS
Hanging Leg Raise	3	12
Lying Leg Raise	3	12
Scissor Kick	3	12

FOREARMS

GRIP-STRENGTH WORKOUT IN FOCUS

Possessing big forearms is a great aesthetic for a man, but superior grip strength will help you in everything from Olympic lifts to sports to life-saving tactics like those a firefighter would need. In this workout, keeping constant tension on the forearms with isometric holds is the method of choice. For 10-pound-plate pinches, hold two plates together in each hand down at your sides for as long as possible. On fat-bar holds, simply hold a heavy, extra-thick barbell (or a standard barbell with a towel wrapped around it) at arm's length in front of your thighs without letting it actually touch you. Again, do this for as long as you can.

GRIP STRENGTH

EXERCISE	SETS	REPS
Wrist Roller	3	Up/Down
10-pound Plate Pinch	3	To failure
Fat-bar Hold	3	To failure

BEHIND-THE-BACK WRIST CURL

To maximize range of motion for full forearm muscle contraction, visualize pulling the weight up so the back of your hands come parallel to the floor.

REVERSE CURL

Reverse curls target the brachioradialis muscle on the outside of the arm near the elbow and the brachialis, which overlaps the biceps.

LIFTING LOWDOWN

A strong pair of forearms will benefit you in many big pushing and pulling exercises because of your increased grip strength. It's important to train your forearms through wrist flexion, extension, and isometric grip holds.

SPLIT DECISION

The forearms can be trained with any number of body parts, most commonly biceps. Just be sure to train them last in your workout since tired forearms will negatively affect most exercises.

REVERSE CURL

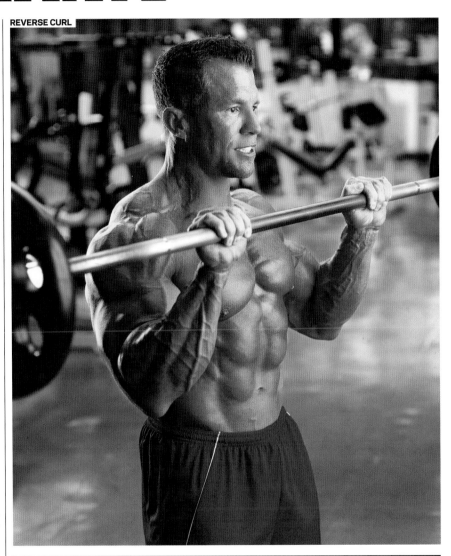

MASS-BUILDING

EXERCISE	SETS	REPS
Wrist Roller	3	Up/Down
Wrist Curl	4	12
Behind-the-back Wrist Curl	4	12

BEGINNER'S

EXERCISE	SETS	REPS
Wrist Roller	3	Up/Down
Reverse Curl	3	10
Wrist Curl	3	10

AT-HOME

EXERCISE	SETS	REPS
Dumbbell Wrist Curl	4	15
Dumbbell Reverse Wrist Curl	4	15
Dumbbell Behind-the-back Wrist Curl	4	15

CALVES

MASS-BUILDING WORKOUT IN FOCUS

It doesn't get much simpler than this workout—three of the most common calf exercises, each performed with the same number of sets and reps—and that's exactly the point. Building up the calves isn't a matter of creativity, it's a matter of sheer doggedness with high volume and relatively high reps, especially if your calves are a stubborn body part. Standing calf raises will add size to the gastrocnemius, while seated calf raises beef up the soleus to cover all bases. Feel free to substitute donkey calf raises for leg-press raises every other workout.

MASS-BUILDING

EXERCISE	SETS	REPS
Standing Calf Raise	4	20
Seated Calf Raise	4	20
Leg-press Calf Raise	4	20

DONKEY CALF RAISE

Don't limit your calf work to standing and seated raises. Maximize training angles and muscle recruitment with variations like donkey calf raises.

SEATED CALF RAISE

Calf exercises in which your knees are bent target the soleus (which lies under the gastrocnemius) to add thickness to the calves.

LIFTING LOWDOWN

The biggest calf-training error is going too heavy and not utilizing a full range of motion on calf raises. Lower your heels until you feel a good stretch in your calves, then press up onto your toes at the top of every rep. If this means you have to use a lighter weight, do it.

SPLIT DECISION

Calves can be trained with any body part and can handle being worked just about every day. Hit your calves at the end of the workout or between exercises for other muscles.

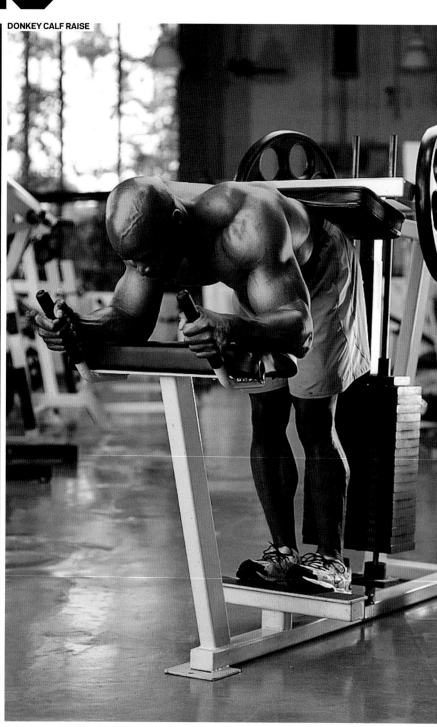

DONKEY CALF RAISE

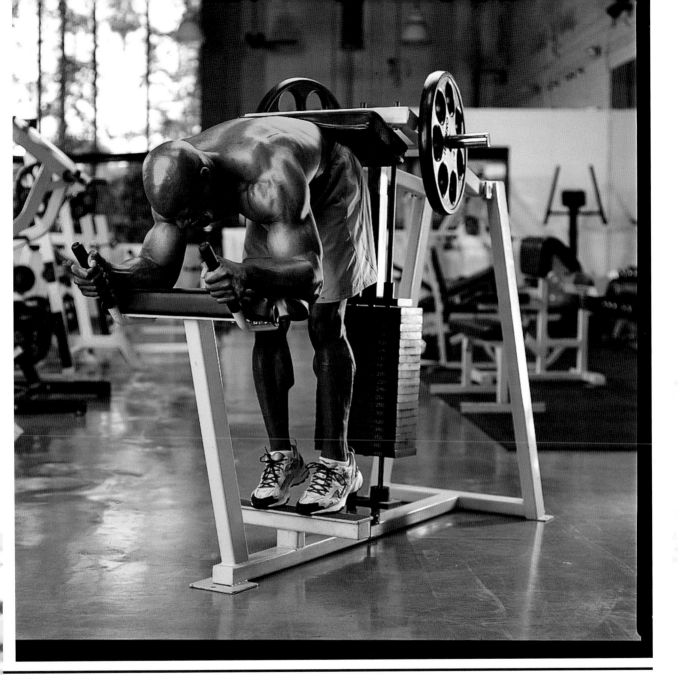

BEGINNER'S		
EXERCISE	SETS	REPS
Standing Calf Raise	3	20
Seated Calf Raise	3	20

AT-HOME		
EXERCISE	SETS	REPS
Standing Dumbbell Calf Raise	4	15
Standing One-leg Dumbbell Calf Raise	4	15 each side

CIRCUIT		
EXERCISE	SETS	REPS
Standing Calf Raise	4	10
Seated Calf Raise	4	10
Donkey Calf Raise	4	10
Pongo Jump On Toes	4	40

Do one set of each movement without resting. Perform the circuit four times, resting one to two minutes between each round.

HAMSTRINGS

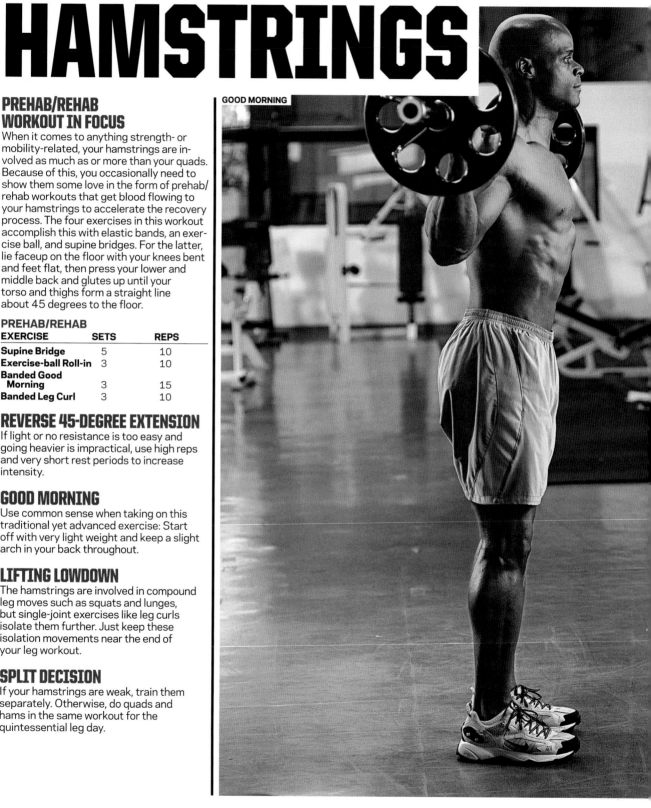

GOOD MORNING

PREHAB/REHAB WORKOUT IN FOCUS

When it comes to anything strength- or mobility-related, your hamstrings are involved as much as or more than your quads. Because of this, you occasionally need to show them some love in the form of prehab/rehab workouts that get blood flowing to your hamstrings to accelerate the recovery process. The four exercises in this workout accomplish this with elastic bands, an exercise ball, and supine bridges. For the latter, lie faceup on the floor with your knees bent and feet flat, then press your lower and middle back and glutes up until your torso and thighs form a straight line about 45 degrees to the floor.

PREHAB/REHAB

EXERCISE	SETS	REPS
Supine Bridge	5	10
Exercise-ball Roll-in	3	10
Banded Good Morning	3	15
Banded Leg Curl	3	10

REVERSE 45-DEGREE EXTENSION

If light or no resistance is too easy and going heavier is impractical, use high reps and very short rest periods to increase intensity.

GOOD MORNING

Use common sense when taking on this traditional yet advanced exercise: Start off with very light weight and keep a slight arch in your back throughout.

LIFTING LOWDOWN

The hamstrings are involved in compound leg moves such as squats and lunges, but single-joint exercises like leg curls isolate them further. Just keep these isolation movements near the end of your leg workout.

SPLIT DECISION

If your hamstrings are weak, train them separately. Otherwise, do quads and hams in the same workout for the quintessential leg day.

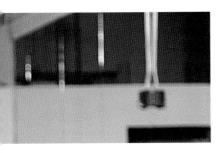

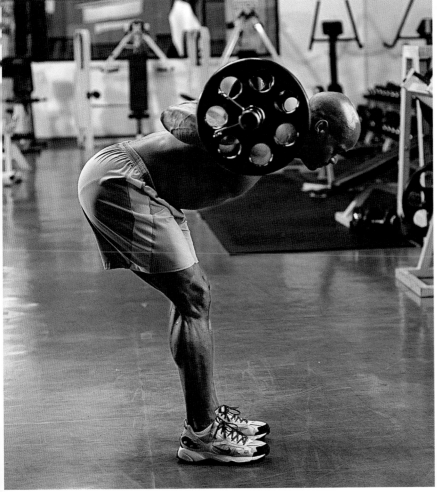

MASS-BUILDING

EXERCISE	SETS	REPS
Deadlift	4	8
Good Morning	3	10
Glute-ham Raise	3	To failure
Leg Curl	3	15

BEGINNER'S

EXERCISE	SETS	REPS
Dumbbell Deadlift	3	8
Exercise-ball Roll-in	3	10
Leg Curl	3	10

AT-HOME

EXERCISE	SETS	REPS
Banded Leg Curl	3	15
Dumbbell Deadlift	3	10
Dumbbell Swing	3	10

15-MINUTE

EXERCISE	SETS	REPS
Romanian Deadlift	3	20
45-degree Back Extension	3	15
Leg Curl	3	20

UPPER/LOWER HAMSTRING PRIORITY

EXERCISE	SETS	REPS
Glute-ham Raise	3	To failure
Reverse 45-degree Extension	3	15
Straight-leg Romanian Deadlift	3	10
Dumbbell Swing	3	10

UNILATERAL-ISOLATION PRIORITY

EXERCISE	SETS	REPS
One-leg Dumbbell Romanian Deadlift	3	10 each side
One-leg Standing Leg Curl	3	12 each side
One-leg Lying Leg Curl	3	12 each side
One-leg 45-degree Back Extension	3	8 each side

STRENGTH/POWER

EXERCISE	SETS	REPS
Deadlift	5	5
Good Morning	5	6
Glute-ham Raise	3	To failure
Dumbbell Snatch	4	6

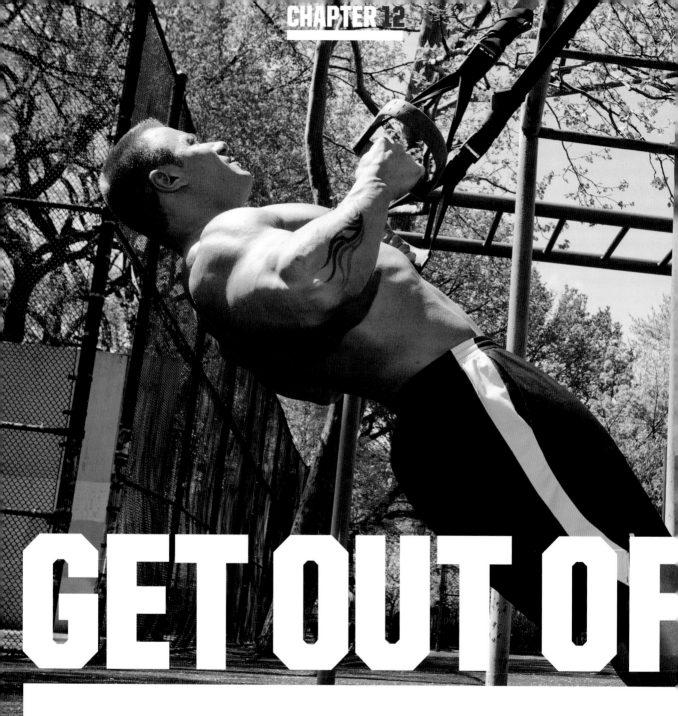

CHAPTER 12

GET OUT OF

TRAIN IN THE GREAT OUTDOORS AND GET RIPPED WITHOUT WEIGHTS

BY JON HINDS, C.N.T.

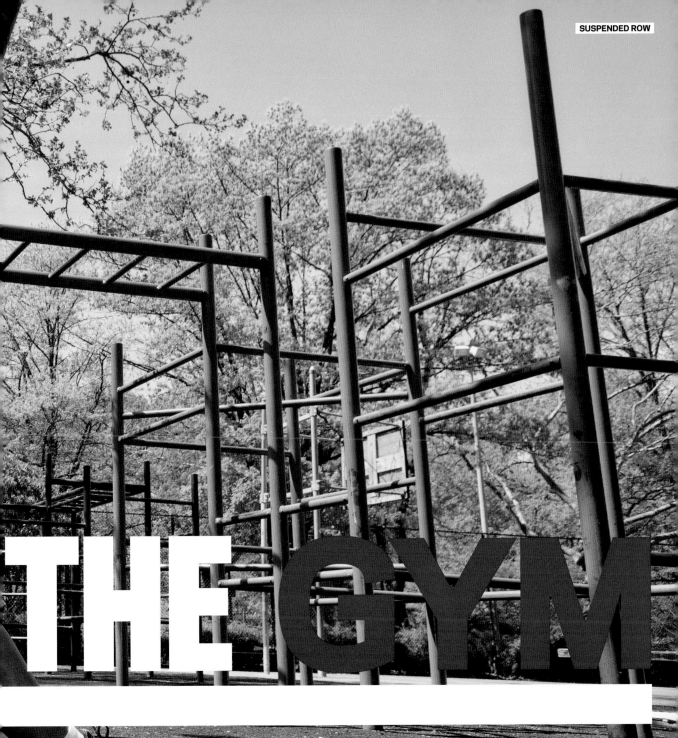

THE GYM

I don't like to lift weights. I'd much rather train outdoors whenever possible. Taking my workouts outside lets me be in the sun (a great way to get vitamin D naturally) and practice all the basic movement skills the way they were intended, using body weight alone. As the founder of Monkey Bar Gymnasiums, a franchise that uses mainly body-weight training to achieve fitness goals, my workouts focus on the activities humans were designed to do to stay healthy, strong, and muscular—that is, running, jumping, crawling, and climbing. No barbells required. And you know what? Even though my students and I are having fun and treating our workouts like kids' games, we're building muscle faster than we would with weights.

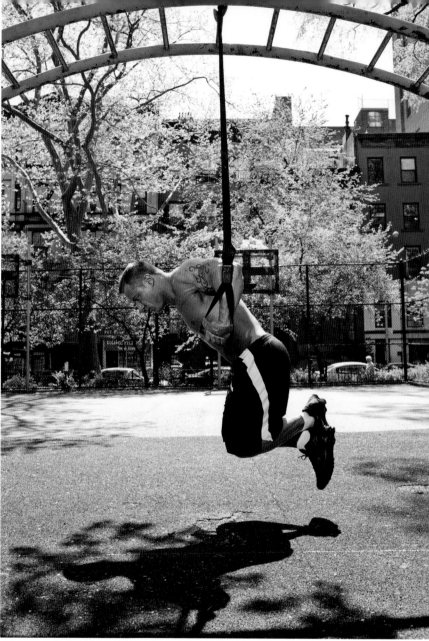

MANY TRAINERS today use body-weight moves only as adjuncts to weight programs—a few sets of pushups at the end of the workout just to finish off the chest, or as a fallback when the trainee has no other equipment available. I think that's very shortsighted, because I've used body-weight training almost exclusively my entire life, and I've gotten results that some lifters never see. When I was in college, a body-weight regimen took my vertical jump from 25 inches to 48. I was hitting my elbow on the rim when I went to dunk. After years of body-weight squats, lunges, jumps, and sprinting, I tried my first deadlift. I pulled 475 for eight reps, easy. Once, I decided to give myself the 225 bench-press test that football players do at the NFL combine. Weighing 205, I did 16 reps, and all I had done for months before were my usual dips and pushup variations.

STRONG AND STABLE

To bench a lot of weight, you need to have a strong connection between your feet and your hands, because as any powerlifter knows, you have to drive your legs into the floor to generate maximum strength when you press. The power travels up from your feet, across your torso, up your arms, and then into the bar. So the tighter you can make every muscle in your body, the stronger the connection and the more force you can produce. The same effect occurs when you do just about any body-weight exercise. First of all, body-weight lifts are closed-chain movements. That means your body is moving around the point where you're applying the force, rather than you moving that point around your body. Think about a dip versus a bench press. When you do a dip, you're moving your whole body around the bars, rather than just moving a barbell off your chest. That makes your central nervous system call in a lot more muscle fibers overall (unless of course you're going for a new max on the bench, in which case you're going to have to give it all you have). Also, while you may only be thinking about training your chest and triceps during a dip, your core has to stay braced to keep your torso from going limp or your legs from swinging during the movement. Your upper back acts like a stabilizer as well. So, getting strong on body-weight pushing moves like the dip teaches your muscles to work as a unit; and, indirectly, they can make you a better bencher.

TAKE THE GYM WITH YOU

I want you to take advantage of warm weather whenever possible and enjoy your training. This program is meant to be done outdoors at a park or playground.

You won't need much equipment—a pullup bar or a strong tree limb, a picnic table, and plenty of open space are enough to get in stellar shape. That said, one of the knocks against body-weight training is that it's hard to progress. For instance, maybe lunges are a joke to you, but you can't do a single-leg squat without falling backward. That's where having some light equipment comes in handy. I've invented a whole line of easy-to-use tools that make body-weight moves adjustable to any skill level. I suggest you pick them up—they'll make the exercises you struggle with easier to

master, and add a new challenge to the ones you think you've already conquered. Your main go-to gadget will be the Jungle Gym XT, a suspension unit. It's the barbell of body-weight training. Use it to adjust your leverage for both upper- and lower-body exercises. When it comes to progressing pushups, the Power Pushup 3 uses cables for resistance. For direct ab training, you can't beat the Power Wheel. Finally, the Power Jumper is essential for developing an explosive lower body. Learn to jump with it, and jumping without it will feel as though you've broken free from gravity.

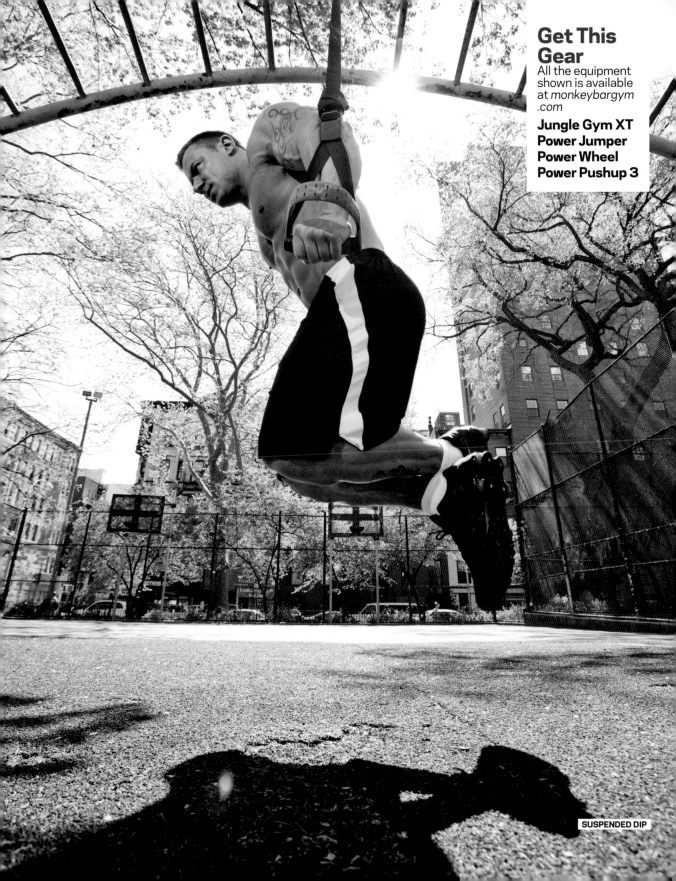

Get This Gear
All the equipment shown is available at *monkeybargym .com*

Jungle Gym XT
Power Jumper
Power Wheel
Power Pushup 3

SUSPENDED DIP

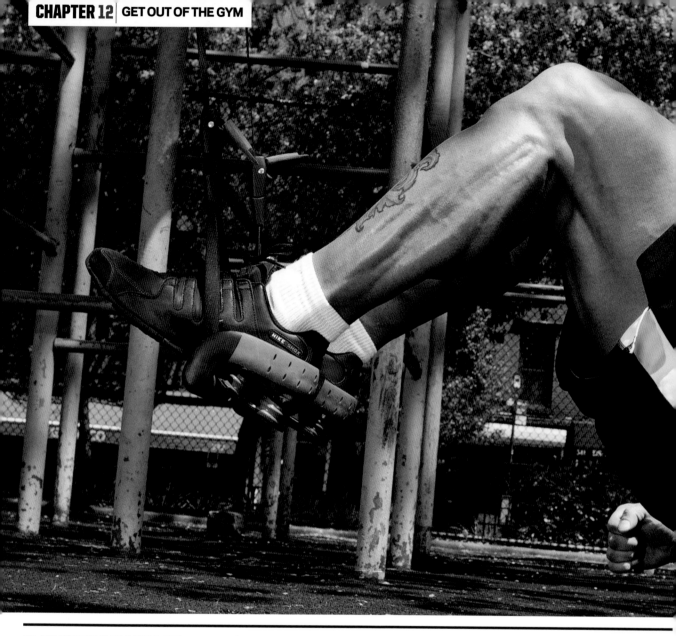

DAY 1 WORKOUT

1A SUSPENDED DIP

Attach a suspension apparatus to a pullup bar. Lower the handles to hip level, and grab ahold. Lower your body until your upper arms are parallel to the ground.

1B L-SIT CHINUP

Bend your hips 90 degrees and extend your legs straight in front of you as you perform each chinup.

2A RESISTED SQUAT TO BOX JUMP

Find a surface about 18 inches above the ground. Attach a resistance band around the back of your neck and feet. Squat down until your fingers touch the ground, then jump up onto the surface. Step back down, and repeat.

2B SUSPENDED LEG CURL

Attach a suspension trainer (such as the Jungle Gym XT, as shown here) to an object overhead—a pullup bar or tree limb will work—and lower the foot stirrups to a few inches above the ground. Lie down on the ground and place your feet in the stirrups. Lift up your hips, then bend your knees and perform a leg curl motion. Keep your hips extended up and off the ground throughout the set.

3 AB ROLLOUT

Hold an ab wheel and rest on your knees (or straighten your legs, as shown, for a greater challenge) a few feet away from a post, tree, or other object. The wheel should be in front of your shoulders. Keeping your abs and hamstrings braced, roll forward about one yard until the post stops the wheel. Roll back.

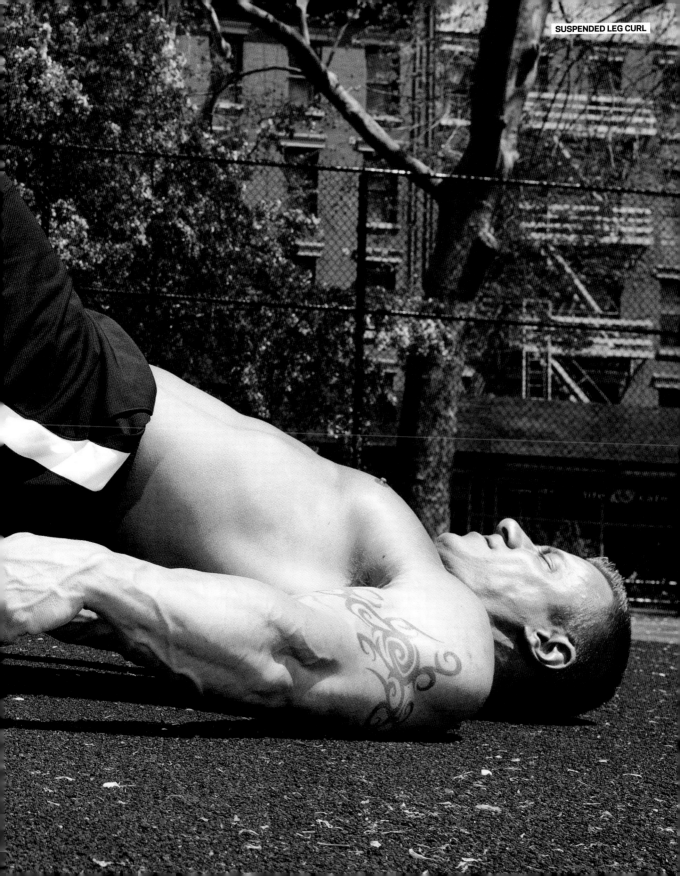

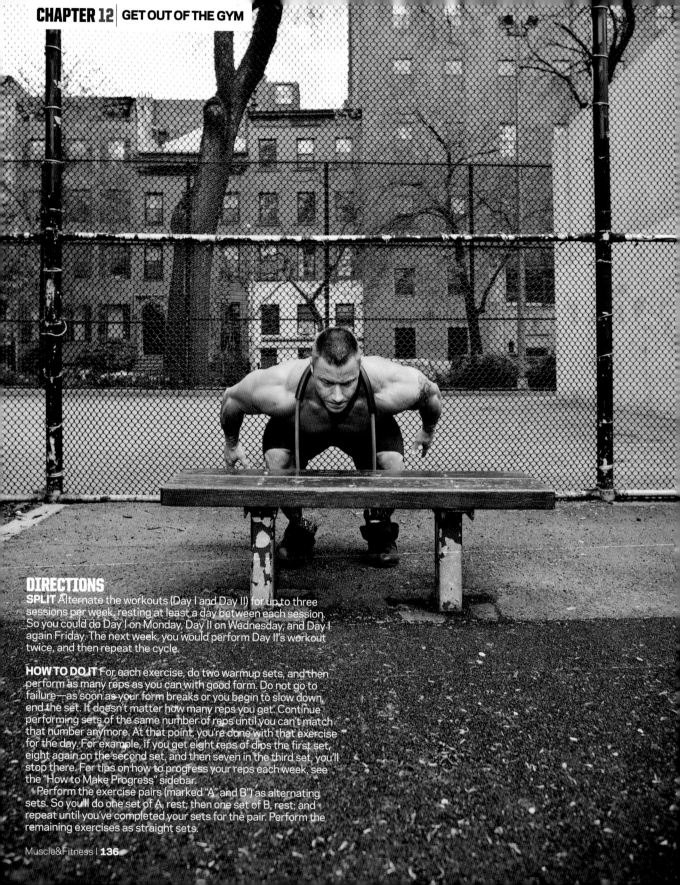

DIRECTIONS

SPLIT Alternate the workouts (Day I and Day II) for up to three sessions per week, resting at least a day between each session. So you could do Day I on Monday, Day II on Wednesday, and Day I again Friday. The next week, you would perform Day II's workout twice, and then repeat the cycle.

HOW TO DO IT For each exercise, do two warmup sets, and then perform as many reps as you can with good form. Do not go to failure—as soon as your form breaks or you begin to slow down, end the set. It doesn't matter how many reps you get. Continue performing sets of the same number of reps until you can't match that number anymore. At that point, you're done with that exercise for the day. For example, if you get eight reps of dips the first set, eight again on the second set, and then seven in the third set, you'll stop there. For tips on how to progress your reps each week, see the "How to Make Progress" sidebar.

Perform the exercise pairs (marked "A" and "B") as alternating sets. So you'll do one set of A, rest; then one set of B, rest; and repeat until you've completed your sets for the pair. Perform the remaining exercises as straight sets.

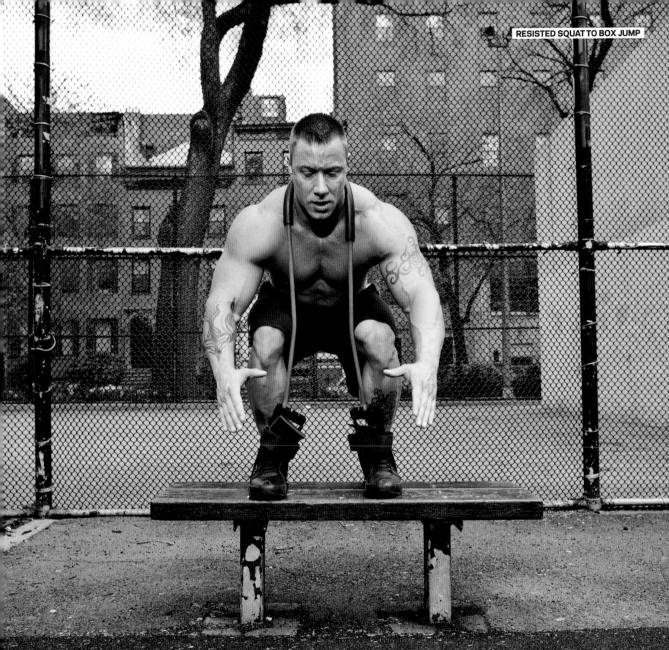

HOW TO MAKE PROGRESS

You're bound to hit a plateau if you make one simple mistake: training too hard. Seriously, trying to increase your reps on every exercise, every time you repeat a workout, is asking too much of your body. Instead, strive to make small weekly improvements on about half of the prescribed moves while you maintain your performance on the rest. After each workout, plan which exercises you'll add a rep to in the next session, and which ones you'll "tie" your reps on. Here's an example of how to plan your training for Day 1's workout. (The first workout is omitted since you'll base your sessions on whatever you can do the first time.) This method will delay a plateau for months.

EXERCISE	2ND WORKOUT	3RD WORKOUT	4TH WORKOUT
Suspended Dip	Add a rep	Same reps as 2nd workout	Add a rep
Chinup	Same reps as 1st workout	Add a rep	Same reps as 3rd workout
Resisted Box Jump	Add a rep	Same reps as 2nd workout	Add a rep
Suspended Leg Curl	Same reps as 1st workout	Add a rep	Same reps as 3rd workout
Ab Rollout	Add a rep	Same reps as 2nd workout	Add a rep

DAY II WORKOUT

1A RESISTED PUSHUP

Wrap a resistance band (or use the Power Pushup 3) around your upper back, and hold an end in each hand. Perform pushups against the resistance, touching your chest to the floor on each rep.

1B SUSPENDED ROW

Attach a suspension apparatus to a pullup bar, tree limb, or other object. Lower the handles, and hang from them so that your torso is parallel to the ground. Squeeze your shoulder blades together and row yourself up.

2A SUSPENDED PISTOL SQUAT TO RUSSIAN LUNGE

Grab the handles of a suspension apparatus, stand on one leg, and raise the other in front of you. Squat down so your butt touches your heel, then come back up. Immediately tuck the free leg behind you, and lower your body again until your knee (but not your foot) touches the floor. That's one rep.

2B GLUTE-HAM RAISE

Kneel on the ground (you can rest your knees on a towel), and brace your heels under a fence or other object that holds them in place. Bend at the hips, and lower your torso as far as you can.

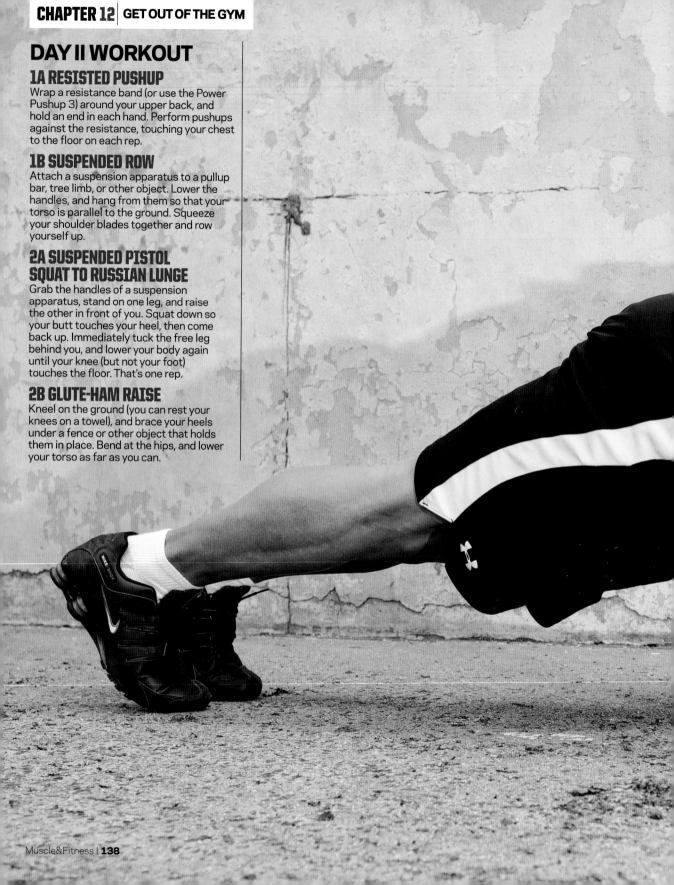

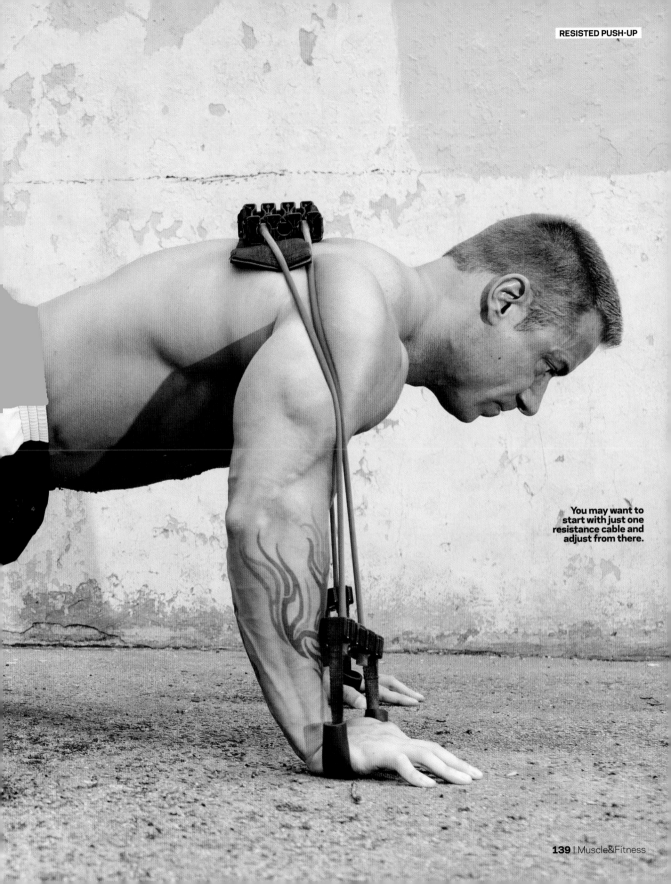

You may want to start with just one resistance cable and adjust from there.

POWER CARDIO

DEVELOP INSANE EXPLOSIVENESS AND GET SHREDDED WITH THIS INTENSE INTERVAL ROUTINE

Here's something you don't see every day: Olympic lifters hosting a fat-burning clinic. We weren't able to get the national weightlifting team to lecture on endurance training, but we did the next best thing: We pulled a page out of the Olympic lifting handbook and applied it to cardio workouts.

It makes total sense because Olympic lifts are full-body exercises that burn a ton of calories and body fat when done for high reps. The explosiveness of the movements is also perfect for ramping up testosterone levels, which leads to a faster metabolism and more muscle mass.

It's like killing two birds with one stone: developing more power, which will help you get bigger and stronger on heavy lifting days; and incinerating body fat through high-intensity, cardio-like intervals, which will help uncover your six-pack. The following Power Cardio program encompasses not only Olympic lifts such as power cleans and snatches but also explosive pushups, lunges, and squats to attack the body from all angles. The only problem: That treadmill you paid top dollar for might collect a little dust in the process.

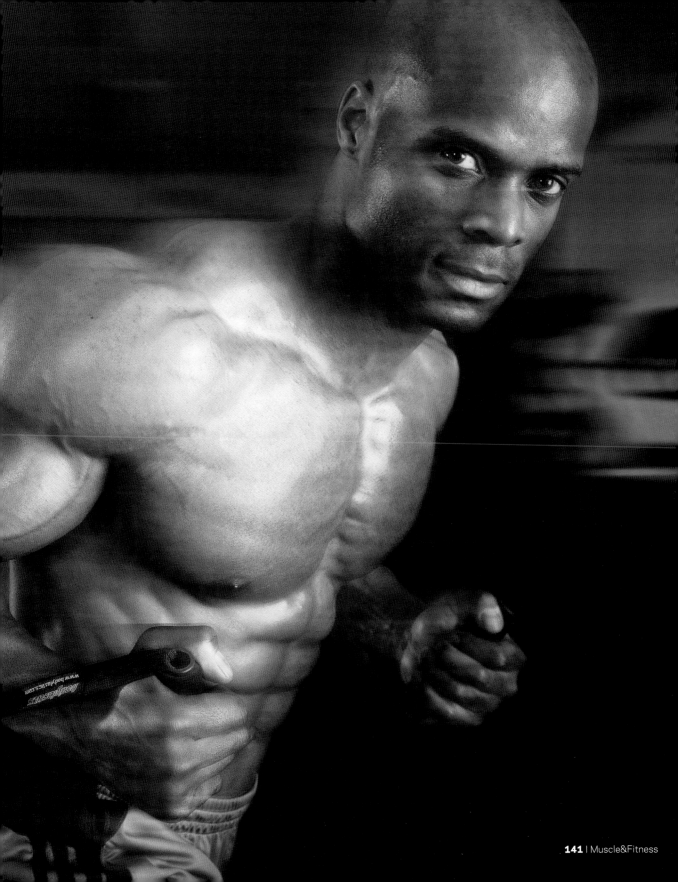

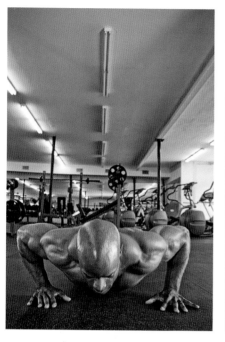
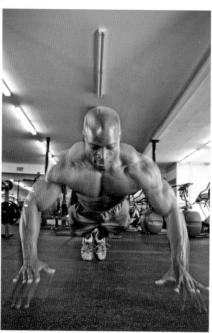
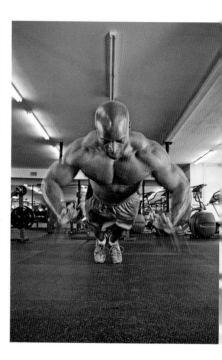

EXPLOSIVE RESULTS

THE KEY TO EFFECTIVELY combining power training and cardio is exercise selection. Isolation moves such as leg extensions and biceps curls have no place here; power-based, compound (multijoint) exercises such as jump squats, cleans, and power pushups are best for recruiting fast-twitch muscle fibers and maximizing fat burning. The explosive nature of the movements is what makes this workout so different from the slow- to moderate-paced reps of traditional bodybuilding programs.

Because of the fast rep speeds, you'll need to keep the weight relatively light. You'll perform many of the exercises in the Power Cardio program using only your body weight, while the rest will incorporate only light dumbbells or barbells. With brief rest periods, heavy lifting is impossible.

The other critical element of Power Cardio is time. This interval-based program alternates 20 seconds of work and rest at a 1:1 work:rest ratio. If the rest periods creep above 20 seconds, you'll lose the workout's cardiovascular and fat-burning benefits. It's imperative that you stick to the intervals, repping out for the full 20 seconds and resuming exactly 20 seconds later.

If the program sounds intense, that's because it is, but volume is kept in check. You'll start with ten 40-second intervals, which will take less than seven minutes to complete. As you get in better shape, you'll add more intervals. In peak condition, you might do as many as 30 intervals in 20 minutes; keep it to 30 to avoid overtraining.

To start, pick five movements and do two sets of each. As you progress, either add exercises or simply do more sets for each move. Perform Power Cardio workouts two to four days per week, either after your regular training split—except on leg days, since most of these exercises are leg-based—or in a separate workout.

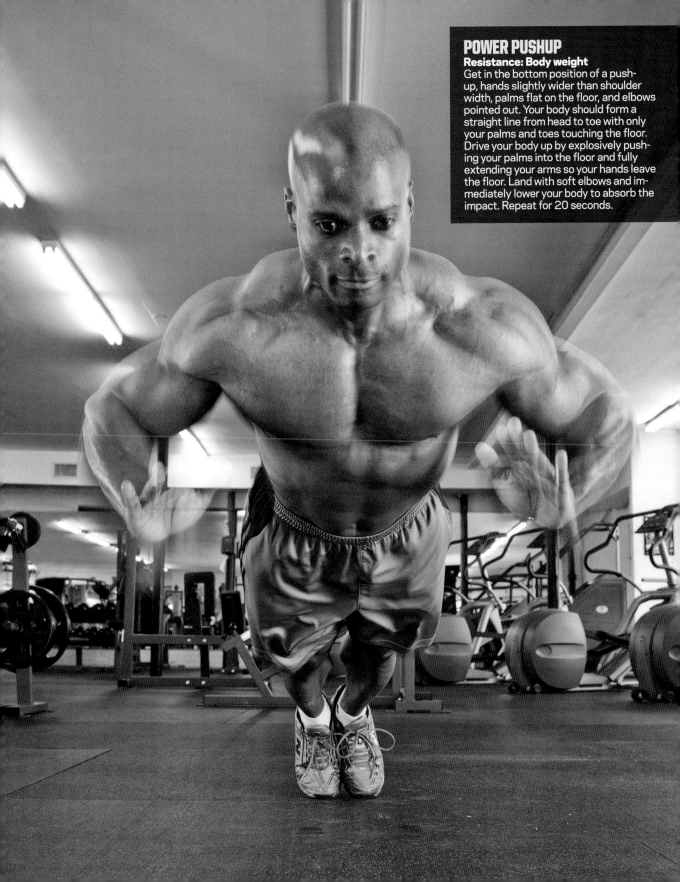

POWER PUSHUP
Resistance: Body weight
Get in the bottom position of a push-up, hands slightly wider than shoulder width, palms flat on the floor, and elbows pointed out. Your body should form a straight line from head to toe with only your palms and toes touching the floor. Drive your body up by explosively pushing your palms into the floor and fully extending your arms so your hands leave the floor. Land with soft elbows and immediately lower your body to absorb the impact. Repeat for 20 seconds.

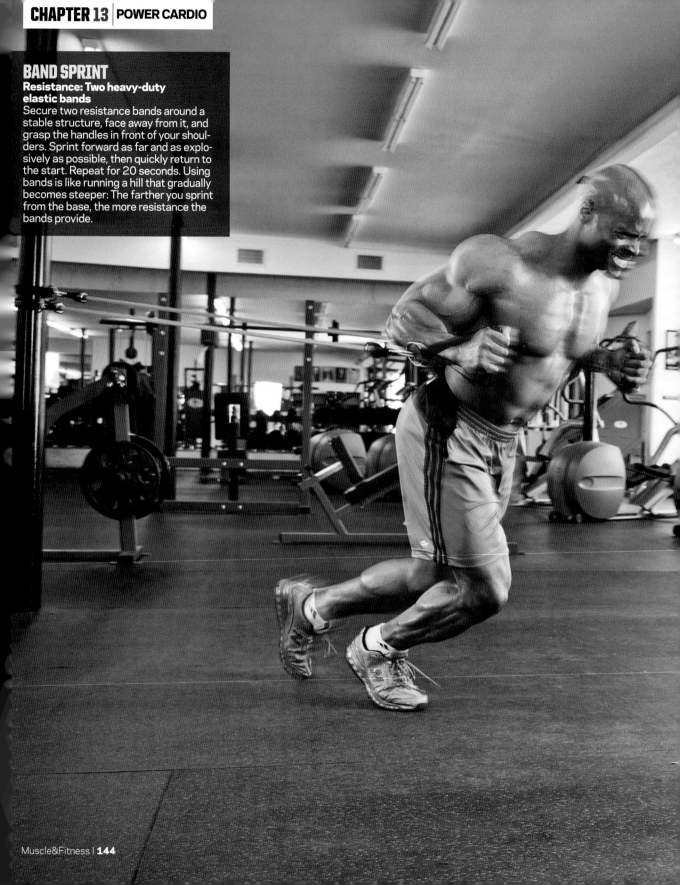

BAND SPRINT

Resistance: Two heavy-duty elastic bands

Secure two resistance bands around a stable structure, face away from it, and grasp the handles in front of your shoulders. Sprint forward as far and as explosively as possible, then quickly return to the start. Repeat for 20 seconds. Using bands is like running a hill that gradually becomes steeper: The farther you sprint from the base, the more resistance the bands provide.

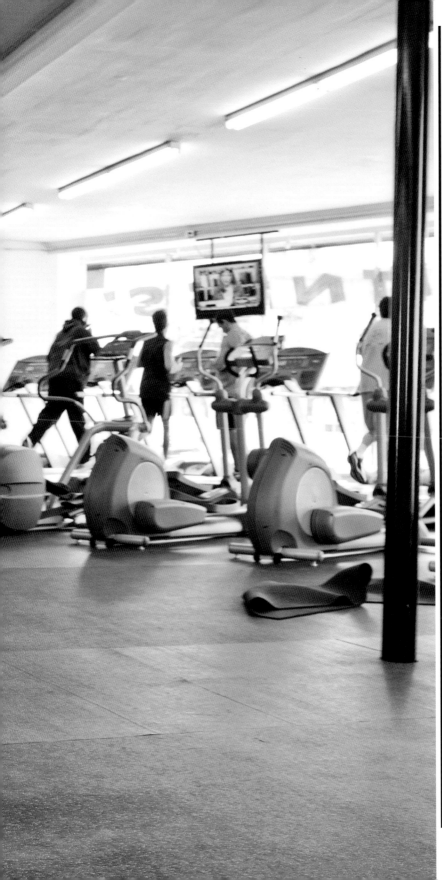

POWER CARDIO ROUTINE

BEGINNER: If you're new to fat-burning cardio workouts based on explosive power exercises, start with two sets of five exercises done two to four days per week as follows:

EXERCISE	SETS	TIME/REST (sec.)
Jump Squat	2	20/20
Band Sprint	2	20/20
Power Pushup	2	20/20
Power Lunge	2	20/20
Power Clean	2	20/20

INTERMEDIATE: As you become more conditioned to Power Cardio workouts, either repeat the above routine for a total of three cycles and/or add exercises. Here's a sample workout:

EXERCISE	SETS	TIME/REST (sec.)
Power Kick-up	2	20/20
One-arm Dumbbell Snatch	2	20/20
Jump Squat	2	20/20
Band Sprint	2	20/20
Power Pushup	2	20/20
Step-up Jump	2	20/20
Power Lunge	2	20/20
Power Clean	2	20/20

ADVANCED: As you progress, add sets until you reach 30 intervals. Stop there to prevent overtraining.

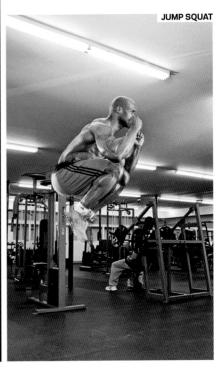

JUMP SQUAT

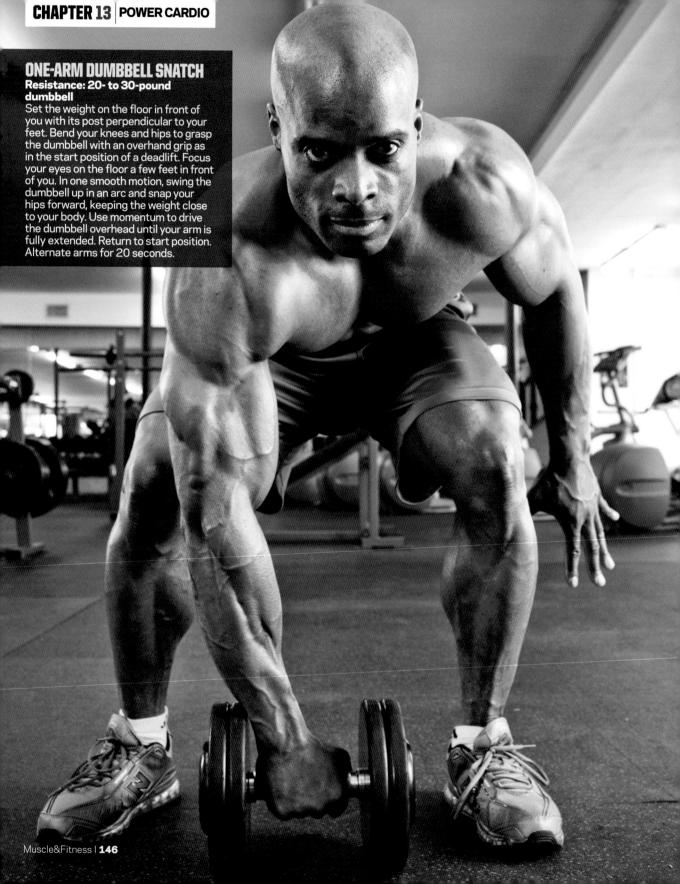

ONE-ARM DUMBBELL SNATCH
Resistance: 20- to 30-pound dumbbell

Set the weight on the floor in front of you with its post perpendicular to your feet. Bend your knees and hips to grasp the dumbbell with an overhand grip as in the start position of a deadlift. Focus your eyes on the floor a few feet in front of you. In one smooth motion, swing the dumbbell up in an arc and snap your hips forward, keeping the weight close to your body. Use momentum to drive the dumbbell overhead until your arm is fully extended. Return to start position. Alternate arms for 20 seconds.

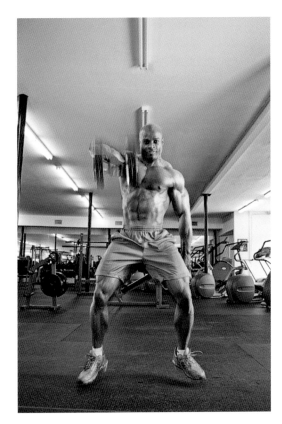
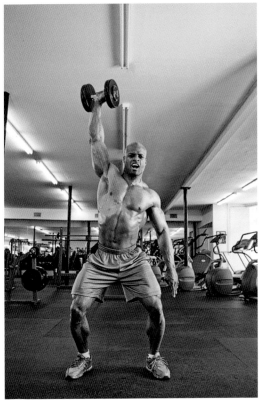

EXERCISES NOT PICTURED

JUMP SQUAT
Resistance: Body weight
Stand erect with your feet about shoulder-width apart, arms by your sides. Maintain the natural arch in your lower back and look forward. Bend your knees and hips, letting your glutes track back, as if to sit in a chair. When your thighs come parallel to the floor, reverse direction, driving up explosively through your heels and the balls of your feet to jump as high as possible. Land with soft knees and immediately descend into the next rep. Repeat for 20 seconds.

STEP-UP JUMP
Resistance: Body weight
Place a knee-level step or bench in front of you and stand erect with your feet hip- to shoulder-width apart. Step onto the platform with one foot and powerfully drive your body up and forward off of it. Land on both feet, knees bent. Turn to face the bench and step up with the opposite leg. Alternate legs for 20 seconds.

POWER LUNGE
Resistance: Light dumbbells or body weight
Stand erect with your feet hip-width apart and head facing forward, and maintain a natural arch in your lower back. Leading with your heel, step forward with your right foot and bend both knees to slowly descend toward the floor. Stop when your left knee almost touches the floor, then explosively push through your right heel, driving yourself back up. Keeping your left foot planted, swing your right leg behind you and stop the momentum by stepping on your right foot. Return to the start position and switch sides. Alternate legs for 20 seconds.

POWER CLEAN
Resistance: Select a weight you can handle for 15-20 reps
Stand erect with your feet shoulder-width apart and your shins about an inch away from a loaded barbell. Squat to grasp the bar with a shoulder-width, overhand grip. With your torso bent 45 degrees over the bar, your arms tensed and pulling on the bar, and your abs pulled in tight, drive explosively through your heels to straighten your knees and bring your hips forward until the bar is at hip level. Immediately lift it, squat under it, and whip your arms around to catch it on your shoulders. Extend your hips and knees to stand erect and rest the bar on your upper chest. Lower the weight to the floor and repeat for 20 seconds.

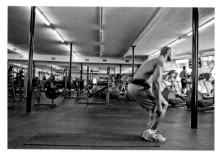

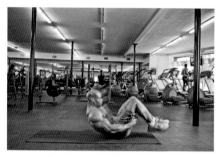

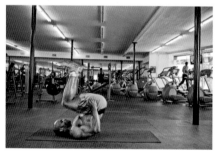

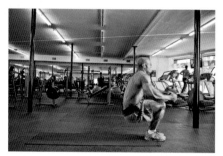

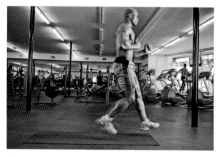

POWER KICK-UP
Resistance: Body weight

Stand erect with your back to a mat and your feet hip- to shoulder-width apart. Squat, then fall back so you land on your glutes. Lean forward and tuck your chin into your chest, then roll onto your upper back and rear delts. Quickly and explosively reverse the motion, using the momentum to plant your feet on the floor and lift yourself off the mat. Explode upward by extending your knees and hips to jump up and back. Land softly with your knees slightly bent. Return to the start and repeat for 20 seconds.

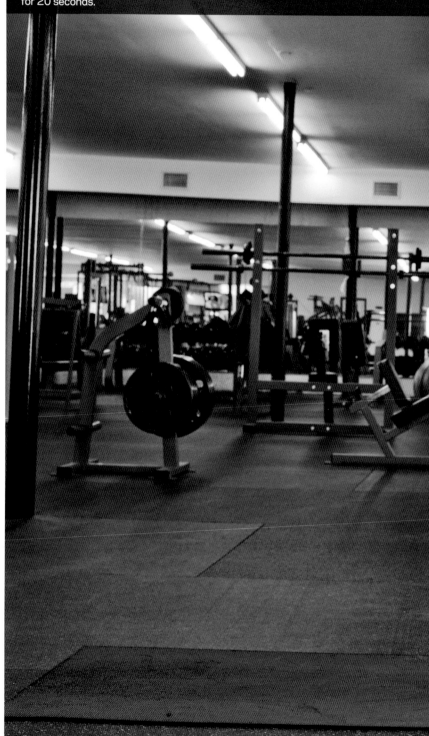

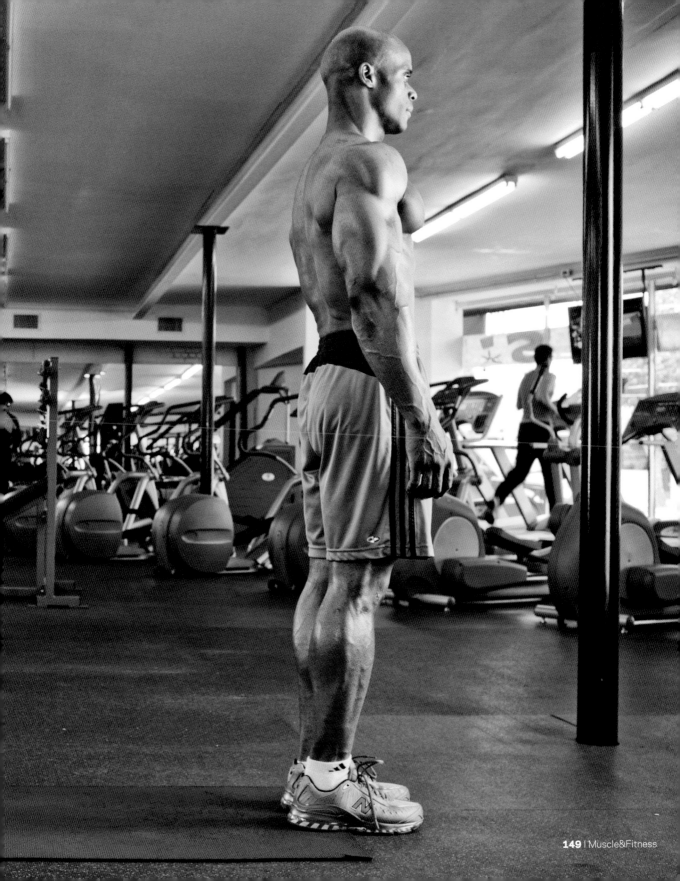

CHAPTER 14

THE A TEAM

WE ASKED 10 OF THE WORLD'S TOP TRAINERS FOR THEIR FAVORITE AB EXERCISE. HERE'S WHAT THEY SAID.

Strengthen your core. These three words have been drilled into athletes and regular gym-goers alike for the better part of a decade, and the wisdom behind them is decidedly sound. Your body is essentially split into halves—upper and lower—but if you lack a solid set of muscles to hold them together and allow them to work in concert, you won't look or perform your best.

The task at hand, then, is figuring out how to train your abdominal muscles in creative and efficient ways that'll enhance both upper- and lower-body development. Most people know just a few boring and repetitive ab exercises, the majority of which contain the words *situp* and *crunch* in their names.

To remedy this, we enlisted 10 of the top names in the fitness industry—handpicked from several different performance genres—to tell us their favorite ab exercises and explain the right ways to do them. Add the moves in this list to your toolbox and watch your midsection transform from weakness to weapon in record time.

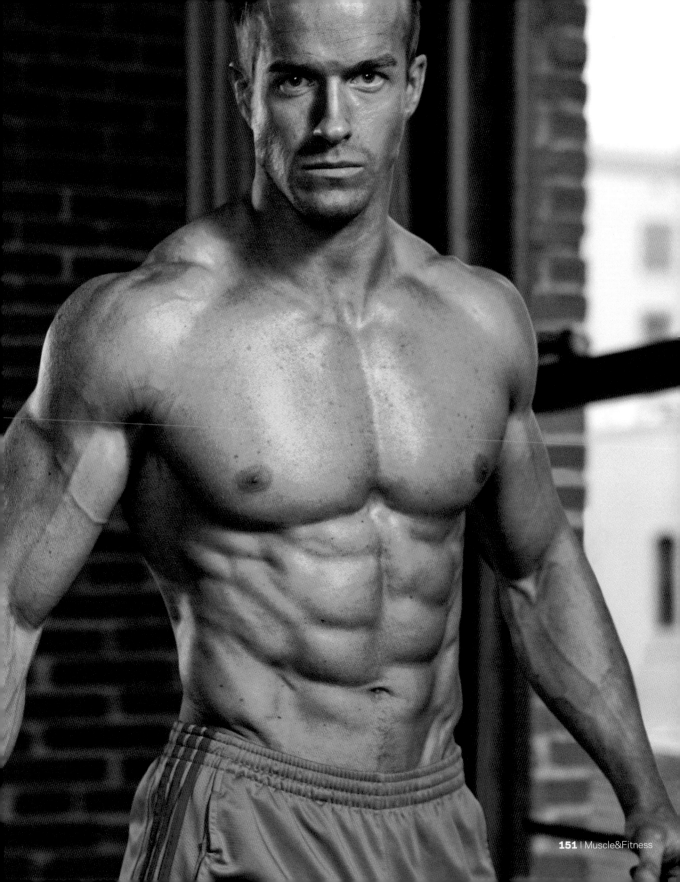

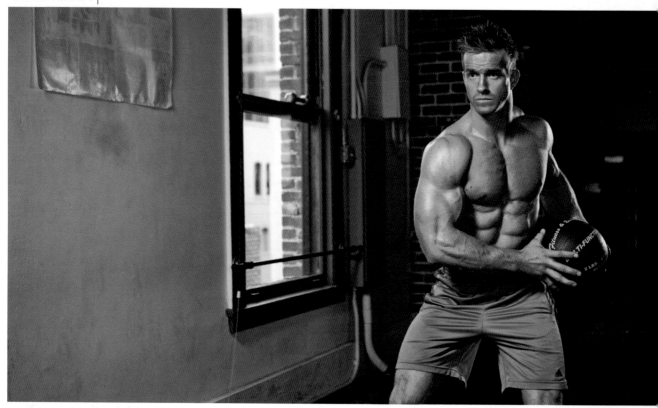

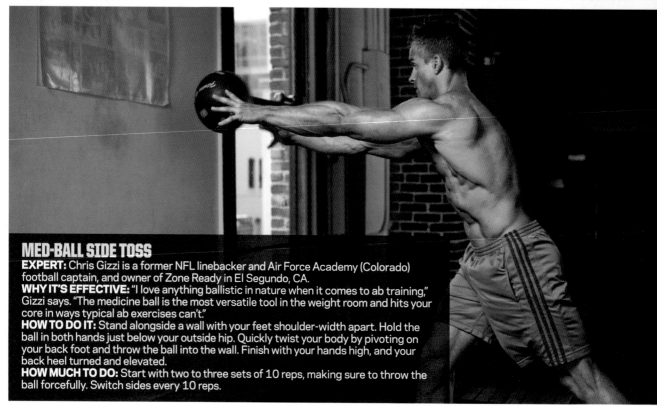

MED-BALL SIDE TOSS

EXPERT: Chris Gizzi is a former NFL linebacker and Air Force Academy (Colorado) football captain, and owner of Zone Ready in El Segundo, CA.

WHY IT'S EFFECTIVE: "I love anything ballistic in nature when it comes to ab training," Gizzi says. "The medicine ball is the most versatile tool in the weight room and hits your core in ways typical ab exercises can't."

HOW TO DO IT: Stand alongside a wall with your feet shoulder-width apart. Hold the ball in both hands just below your outside hip. Quickly twist your body by pivoting on your back foot and throw the ball into the wall. Finish with your hands high, and your back heel turned and elevated.

HOW MUCH TO DO: Start with two to three sets of 10 reps, making sure to throw the ball forcefully. Switch sides every 10 reps.

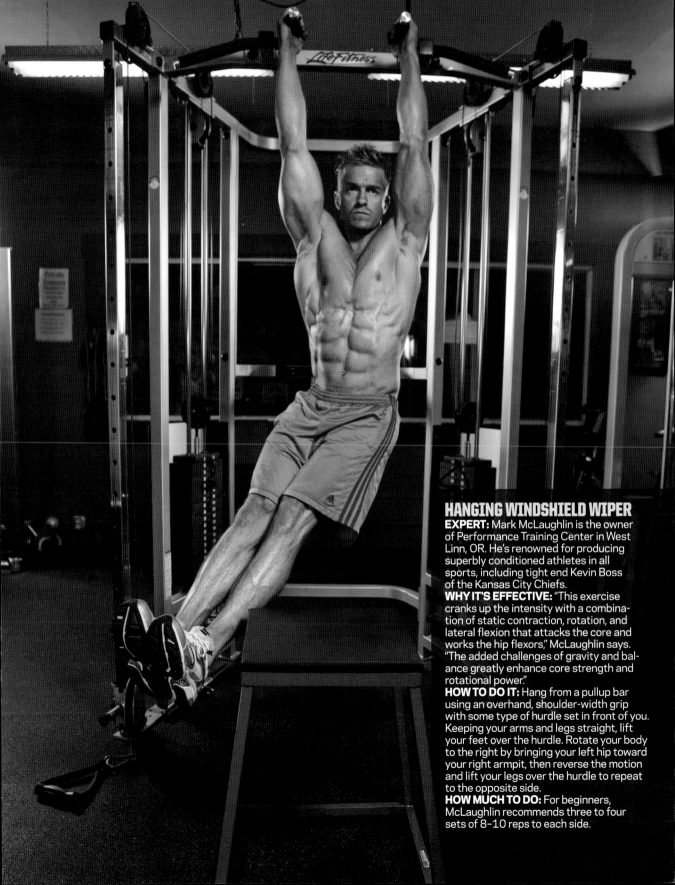

HANGING WINDSHIELD WIPER

EXPERT: Mark McLaughlin is the owner of Performance Training Center in West Linn, OR. He's renowned for producing superbly conditioned athletes in all sports, including tight end Kevin Boss of the Kansas City Chiefs.

WHY IT'S EFFECTIVE: "This exercise cranks up the intensity with a combination of static contraction, rotation, and lateral flexion that attacks the core and works the hip flexors," McLaughlin says. "The added challenges of gravity and balance greatly enhance core strength and rotational power."

HOW TO DO IT: Hang from a pullup bar using an overhand, shoulder-width grip with some type of hurdle set in front of you. Keeping your arms and legs straight, lift your feet over the hurdle. Rotate your body to the right by bringing your left hip toward your right armpit, then reverse the motion and lift your legs over the hurdle to repeat to the opposite side.

HOW MUCH TO DO: For beginners, McLaughlin recommends three to four sets of 8–10 reps to each side.

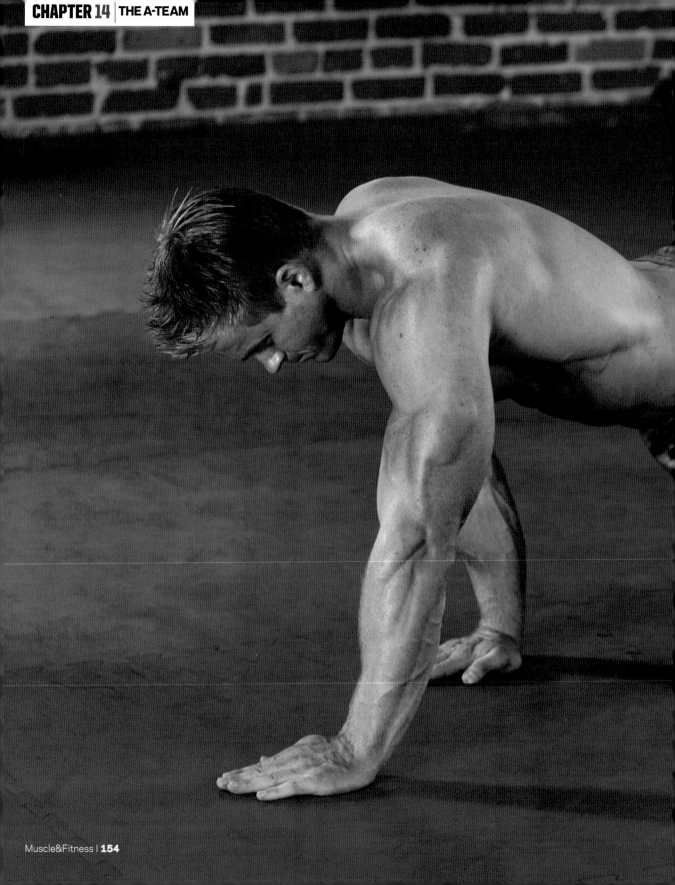

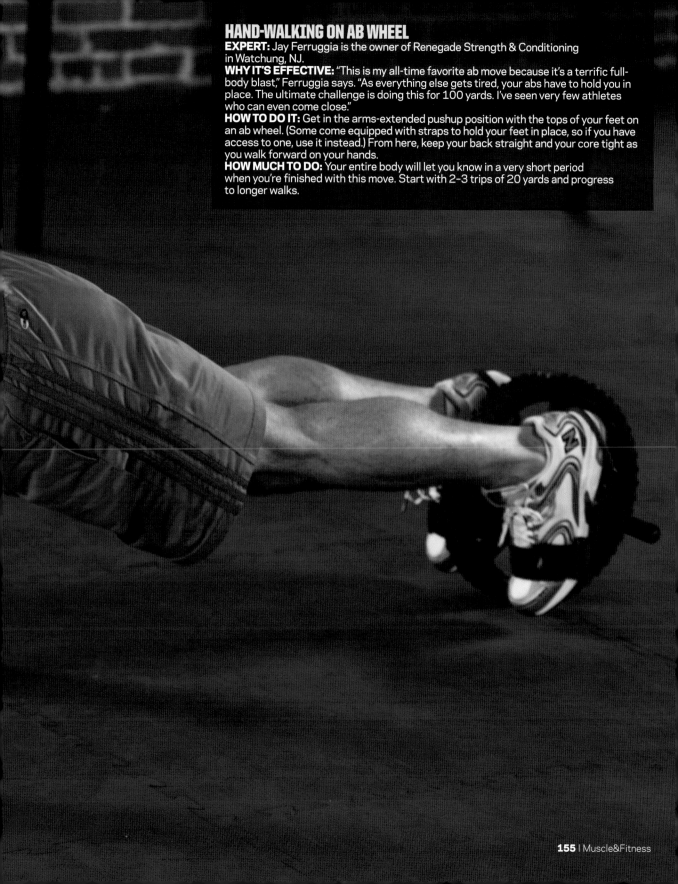

HAND-WALKING ON AB WHEEL

EXPERT: Jay Ferruggia is the owner of Renegade Strength & Conditioning in Watchung, NJ.

WHY IT'S EFFECTIVE: "This is my all-time favorite ab move because it's a terrific full-body blast," Ferruggia says. "As everything else gets tired, your abs have to hold you in place. The ultimate challenge is doing this for 100 yards. I've seen very few athletes who can even come close."

HOW TO DO IT: Get in the arms-extended pushup position with the tops of your feet on an ab wheel. (Some come equipped with straps to hold your feet in place, so if you have access to one, use it instead.) From here, keep your back straight and your core tight as you walk forward on your hands.

HOW MUCH TO DO: Your entire body will let you know in a very short period when you're finished with this move. Start with 2-3 trips of 20 yards and progress to longer walks.

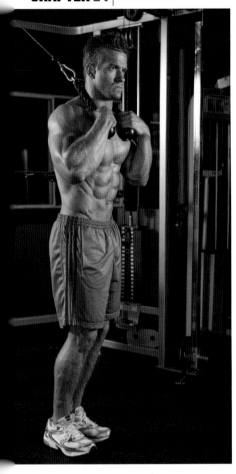

STANDING CABLE CRUNCH

EXPERT: Dave Tate is a former world-class powerlifter, consultant to collegiate and professional sports programs, and owner of Elite Fitness Systems in London, OH.

WHY IT'S EFFECTIVE: "I love this move for strength athletes because it stretches and opens the hips," Tate says. "When you can't control your hips, you can't squat with authority or drive your glutes forward to finish a deadlift."

HOW TO DO IT: Stand facing away from a high-pulley cable station with your feet shoulder-width apart and your knees slightly bent. Grasp a rope attachment with both hands and pull it around your neck, holding it against your chest. Bend at the waist and crunch forward until your forearms touch your thighs, then return to the start.

HOW MUCH TO DO: Tate recommends a high volume of reps with this move. Start with sets of 20 or timed sets of two minutes.

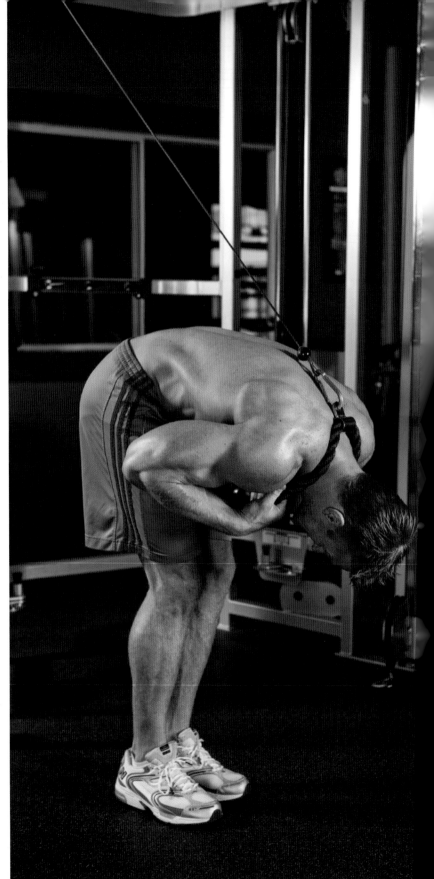

SITUP TO STANDING

EXPERT: Cornell Key is a former All-American defensive end at Monmouth University in New Jersey and owner of Key2 Sports & Fitness, where he trains college and professional athletes.

WHY IT'S EFFECTIVE: "This is a dynamic movement that adds an element of explosiveness to conventional situps," Key says. "The transition to a standing position mimics the kind of core exertion athletes need in competition."

HOW TO DO IT: Lie faceup with your knees bent, holding a dumbbell or plate at your chest with both hands. Forcefully bend at the waist, pull your heels slightly back toward your glutes and explosively stand up. From a standing position, carefully descend into a squat, roll your torso back to the start and rhythmically begin your next rep.

HOW MUCH TO DO: "This isn't an easy exercise to master, so start with modest expectations," Key says. "Three sets of five reps or so should be fine for beginners."

ROMAN-CHAIR SITUP

EXPERT: Matt Kroczaleski is a world-class powerlifter who has squatted 1,014 pounds and deadlifted 810 at a bodyweight of 242 pounds.

WHY IT'S EFFECTIVE: "This exercise is a compound movement that forces you to flex your abs really hard to maintain stability," Kroczaleski says. "It also works your hip flexors. That's the kind of strength you need when you're under an incredibly heavy squat."

HOW TO DO IT: Position yourself on a roman chair or bench so that when your legs are straight, your waist extends past the pad with your lower legs anchored. Hold a plate at your chest or forehead and slowly lean back using your abs until you're horizontal, suspending yourself by your feet. Crunch your abs to return to the 90-degree upright position.

HOW MUCH TO DO: Start with your body weight for sets of 10, then gradually add weight, keeping your rep range at 6–10 per set.

BARBELL ROLLOUT

EXPERT: Joel Jamieson is the author of *Ultimate MMA Conditioning*, and a strength and conditioning coach to MMA fighters Rich Franklin, Chris Leben and Matt Brown.

WHY IT'S EFFECTIVE: "It's the same exercise you'd do with a little ab wheel, only you can change the height of your hands with a barbell," Jamieson says. "It's a phenomenal overall ab move."

HOW TO DO IT: Place a loaded barbell on the floor—Jamieson likes using either 45- or 25-pound plates—then bend over and grasp it with an overhand, shoulder-width grip. Roll the bar forward and past your head until your body is fully extended, nearly horizontal, and your arms are in line with your body. Then return to the start position.

HOW MUCH TO DO: "This isn't an exercise I'd prescribe for beginners," Jamieson says. "But if you're able to do reps, I'd suggest three sets, stopping one rep shy of failure each time."

EXERCISE-BALL MOUNTAIN CLIMBER

EXPERTS: Shannon Turley is the strength and conditioning coach for the Stanford University football team, and Ross Bowsher is the assistant strength and conditioning coach for Butler University basketball team in Indianapolis.

WHY IT'S EFFECTIVE: "We invest so much in this exercise because it trains the core to run," Turley says. "It serves the dual role of stabilizing the torso, and creating stability in one leg and mobility in the other, coming from the core. If you can't stabilize your core, you can't do it."

HOW TO DO IT: Get in pushup position with your forearms on an exercise ball and your feet together, then drive one knee as high as you can, keeping your shoulder, head, knee and ankle in a straight line. Bring your knee as close to your chest as you can and stabilize your torso with your shoulders.

HOW MUCH TO DO: Bowsher recommends starting with three sets of 10 reps with each knee, then increasing your training volume as you become familiar with the movement.

HANGING LEG RAISE VARIATION

EXPERT: Josh Bryant, C.S.C.S., is a trainer at legendary MetroFlex Gym in Arlington, TX. At 22, he was the youngest man in history to bench-press 600 pounds without supportive equipment.

WHY IT'S EFFECTIVE: "Real life happens all around you, all 360 degrees of it," Bryant says. "But for the sagittal plane—where most training in the gym takes place with squatting, benching, and curls—hanging leg raises with static holds are the best exercise I've found for strengthening the abs."

HOW TO DO IT: Hang from an overhead pullup bar. Keeping your legs straight and feet together, raise your feet to waist level, hold for a second, then spread your legs as far apart as you can. Hold this position for a second, bring your feet back together, then slowly lower to the start.

HOW MUCH TO DO: This is a very difficult exercise to do for reps, so Bryant suggests simply performing three sets to the point where you can no longer use proper form.

DECLINE-BENCH REVERSE CRUNCH

EXPERT: Hany Rambod is the creator of the FST-7 bodybuilding training protocol and trainer to Mr. Olympia winners Jay Cutler and Phil Heath.

WHY IT'S EFFECTIVE: "This movement fires the abs in probably the most effective way possible," Rambod says. "In my experience, it makes you more sore than any other exercise. It hits both the lower and upper abs, especially when you lift your hips toward the ceiling."

HOW TO DO IT: Lie faceup on a decline bench with your head higher than your hips and grasp the top of the bench with your hands above your head. Raise your knees to your elbows as you lift your hips and glutes off the bench. Slowly lower your hips and knees to return to the start position.

HOW MUCH TO DO: For beginners, Rambod recommends multiple sets of 10–15 reps.

CHAPTER 15

FEED YO

UR ABS

YOUR TRAINING WON'T GET YOU CUT IF YOUR DIET IS OUT OF WHACK. THESE 13 SIX-PACK-PROMOTING FOODS NEED TO BE ON YOUR GROCERY LIST.

From now on, you're going to ask yourself one question before you eat any food: "Will it help me build abs?" If your answer is no…well, we won't patronize you. But we've made knowing what to eat simpler by collecting the most abs-friendly foods in the world—a list assembled for us by Ryan Andrews, R.D., C.S.C.S., director of education at Precision Nutrition, a nutrition education company in Toronto. The more of these super-foods you can work into your diet—in no particular order—the leaner you'll get.

KALE

This leafy green is "calorie dilute," meaning it's relatively low in calories for its size and is packed with fiber. Kale is also loaded with minerals, including calcium and iron.

ANDREWS SAYS: *"Getting enough calcium might actually help to regulate appetite, alter how much fat is absorbed into your gut, and improve your cells' ability to use fat as an energy source. When you don't have enough iron in the body, you don't have enough oxygen getting to cells, which leads to unproductive workouts and fatigue."*

NUTRITION FACTS
CHOPPED KALE, 1 CUP
33 calories
2g protein
7g carbs
0g fat
1g fiber

MUSHROOMS

Very low in both total calories and carbs, not to mention it's fat-free, the mushroom's main selling point is that it's a very good source of vitamin D—which has been shown to aid in fat loss as well as boost testosterone and strength levels.

ANDREWS SAYS: *"Nearly every tissue and cell in our body has a vitamin D receptor, and low levels of vitamin D have been associated with loss of muscle, lowered immunity, and lowered insulin sensitivity. Last time I checked, these three things didn't help anyone get a lean body."*

NUTRITION FACTS
RAW WHITE MUSHROOMS, 1 CUP
21 calories
3g protein
3g carbs
0g fat
1g fiber

WALNUTS

The abundance of healthy omega-3 fats in walnuts make it a great snack to tide you over until your next meal. Adding chopped walnuts to a salad or other recipes can instantly turn a carb-centric dish into a more balanced one.

ANDREWS SAYS: *"People tend to do really well from a satiety standpoint when eating whole, raw nuts. You'll feel more satisfied after eating because of the fat content."*

NUTRITION FACTS
WALNUTS, 1 OZ
183 calories
4g protein
4g carbs
18g fat
2g fiber

BRUSSELS SPROUTS

Loaded with vitamins and minerals, Brussels sprouts are one of the best sources of vitamin C you can find. (If you're the type who's avoided them since childhood, we won't ask you to eat them a lot—although you may change your mind if you drizzle them with olive oil, add a dusting of sea salt, and bake.) Sprouts are low in calories but high in fiber.
ANDREWS SAYS: "The frozen kind are just as beneficial."

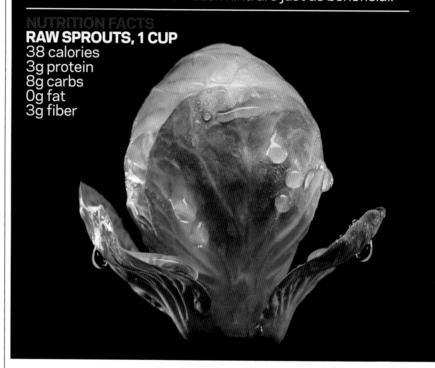

NUTRITION FACTS
RAW SPROUTS, 1 CUP
38 calories
3g protein
8g carbs
0g fat
3g fiber

ROLLED OATS

Yes, oats are carbs, which to some are the abs' ultimate enemy. But oats can be six-pack friendly, thanks to their resistant starch. Most starches get broken down into glucose and, when there's a surplus, are eventually stored as body fat. But not resistant starch. It doesn't get broken down and ends up acting like fiber in the body.

ANDREWS SAYS: *"Because you don't absorb the resistant starch in rolled oats, the food actually has fewer calories than indicated on the label."*

NUTRITION FACTS
DRY OATS, ½ CUP
190 calories
7g protein
32g carbs
3.5g fat
5g fiber

SWEET POTATO

Most starchy carbs should be eaten sparingly when trying to shed body fat because of their effect on insulin levels. When insulin climbs in response to a starch entering the bloodstream, fat burning shuts down. Sweet potatoes are an exception. You're not likely to overeat them due to their fiber and water content. They're also a good source of vitamins A and B6, and minerals manganese and potassium.

ANDREWS SAYS: *"Squash is a great option, too. It's loaded with micronutrients."*

NUTRITION FACTS
SWEET POTATO, 5-INCHES LONG
112 calories
2g protein
26g carbs
0g fat
4g fiber

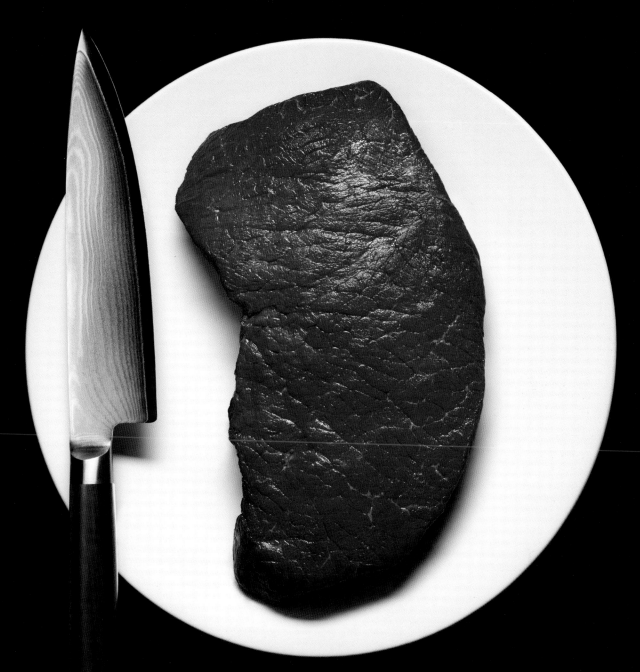

LEAN, GRASS-FED BEEF

Any intense fat-burning training program (like the ones found in this book) will also burn up muscle tissue if you're not getting enough protein in your diet. Grass-fed beef has copious amounts, along with other beneficial ingredients like omega-3s and conjugated linoleic acid (CLA), a chemical that's been linked to fat burning. Cows raised on grass contain more CLA than corn- or grain-fed beef.

ANDREWS SAYS: *"Pasture-raised cows are often healthier than ones raised on factory farms."*

NUTRITION FACTS
TENDERLOIN, 6 OZ
258 calories
36g protein
0g carbs
12g fat
0g fiber

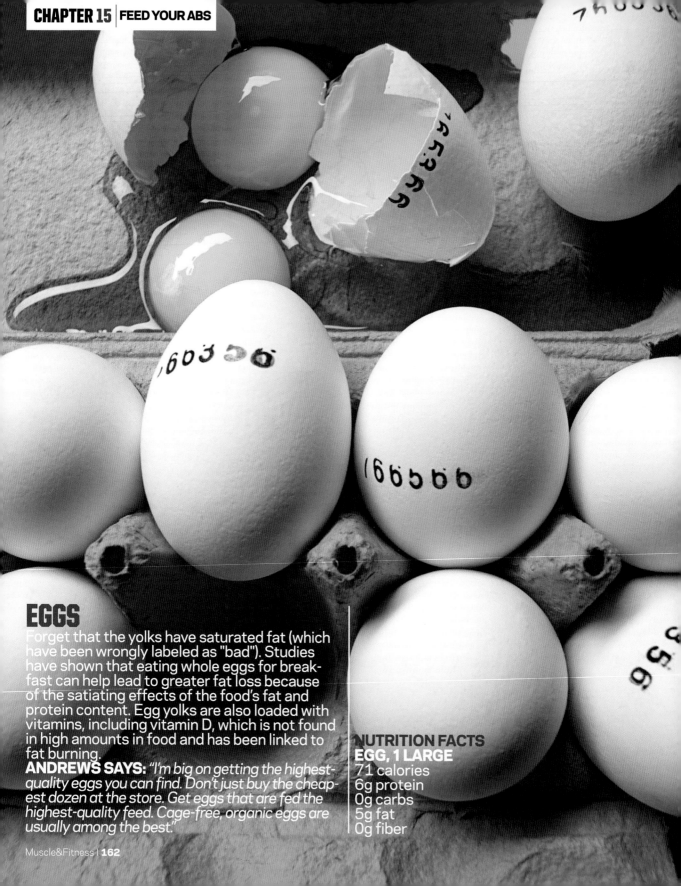

EGGS

Forget that the yolks have saturated fat (which have been wrongly labeled as "bad"). Studies have shown that eating whole eggs for breakfast can help lead to greater fat loss because of the satiating effects of the food's fat and protein content. Egg yolks are also loaded with vitamins, including vitamin D, which is not found in high amounts in food and has been linked to fat burning.

ANDREWS SAYS: *"I'm big on getting the highest-quality eggs you can find. Don't just buy the cheapest dozen at the store. Get eggs that are fed the highest-quality feed. Cage-free, organic eggs are usually among the best."*

NUTRITION FACTS
EGG, 1 LARGE
71 calories
6g protein
0g carbs
5g fat
0g fiber

AVOCADO

The healthy-fat and fiber content in an avocado make it a great fat-burning food for one simple reason: satiety. You'll feel fuller after eating only a small amount, making you less likely to overeat.

ANDREWS SAYS: *"When we eat enough healthy, omega-3 fats over time, they actually become part of our body cells and increase our ability to use body fat as an energy source."*

NUTRITION FACTS
AVOCADO, 1 CUP, SLICED
234 calories
3g protein
12g carbs
21g fat
10g fiber

HEMP SEEDS

This isn't the first food that comes to mind for most people when putting together a get-lean diet, but hemp seeds are loaded with complete protein and are also a decent source of omega-3 fats and fiber. Add these to your next shake, and you're getting great muscle-building benefits on top of satiety.

ANDREWS SAYS: *"Hemp seeds have a nice flavor and offer the full gamut of get-lean ingredients."*

NUTRITION FACTS
HEMP SEEDS, 4 TBSP
320 calories
22g protein
14g carbs
20g fat
2g fiber

WILD SALMON

Salmon is chock-full of nutrients that help you get better abs ASAP—specifically protein, omega-3 fats, vitamin D, and calcium. Like a meal with eggs, dinner built around a salmon fillet will leave you satisfied because it helps build and repair muscles.

ANDREWS SAYS: *"Fish can be unsustainably harvested and contaminated. That's why it's important to choose wild, not farmed, salmon. It's also important to figure out which ocean the fish was caught in, and then make sure that area isn't being overfished."* Andrews recommends checking the Seafood Watch at montereybayaquarium.org *before deciding what type of salmon to purchase. "Cheap seafood is suspect."*

NUTRITION FACTS
WILD ATLANTIC, ½ FILLET, COOKED
280 calories
39g protein
0g carbs
13g fat
0g fiber

DRINK TO THIS:
HERBAL TEA
Calories from beverages are a major abs-killer for those hooked on sugar-filled Starbucks concoctions, energy drinks, and regular soda. Drinking water is always a good option, but where getting a six-pack is concerned, herbal tea is even better. Compounds found in green, white, and black tea are believed to speed up metabolism, even if only slightly, and the calorie reduction from switching over from macchiatos and lattes can measure in the hundreds per day. This way, you don't have to give up your coffee; just make sure to drink it black. Cream and sugar are physique wreckers.

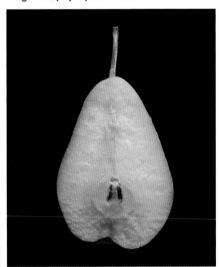

BLACK BEANS

Beans are a great multitasking food in that they provide fiber, are relatively low in calories, and are a good source of protein. Black (or lentil) beans are great in salads or to have on the side with another lean source of protein like lean beef, chicken, or fish.

ANDREWS SAYS: *"They're great for satiety because of the protein and fiber."*

NUTRITION FACTS
BLACK BEANS, ½ CUP, RAW
331 calories
21g protein
60g carbs
3g fat
14g fiber

PEARS

How many people have you known who got fat from eating whole fruits? Zero. Like kale, pears are calorie dilute and rich in fiber. They're ideal for a guy who needs to make every food count while avoiding a calorie surplus.

ANDREWS SAYS: *"You'd have to eat about eight pounds of pears a day to overdo it on calories. It's so tough to overeat them in their whole form. Don't eat them dried—you get more sugar without the filling water."*

NUTRITION FACTS
PEAR, 1 LARGE
133 calories
1g protein
36g carbs
0g fat
7g fiber

FOOD FOR THOUGHT
Nutritionist Ryan Andrews, R.D., C.S.C.S., offers these simple guidelines for getting lean—no calorie-counting required

LISTEN TO HUNGER CUES. Pay attention to what your body tells you. Listen when it says you're hungry and when you're not. If you're kind of hungry, it's probably time to eat. When you're no longer hungry, stop eating. Some guys just load up until they're stuffed, while others let themselves get too hungry during the day, which leads to making bad decisions and overeating later on. Eat just enough to hold you over for a few hours, to keep a nice flow of amino acids to your muscles and keep your metabolism high all day.

EAT PROTEIN AT EVERY MEAL. Though Andrews isn't big on one specific protein-intake recommendation, he advises having protein at every feeding. (M&F recommends at least one gram of protein per pound of body weight per day, even on a fat-burning diet.) Ample protein intake increases satiety and promotes muscle growth and a faster metabolism—all of which will help you maximize leanness.

DON'T RULE OUT CARBS. "I don't recommend going low-carb to get lean, but cut out the crappy carbs (cereal, chips, crackers, etc.)," Andrews says. If your carbs are from whole oats, vegetables, and fruits, you won't store extra fat. "It's tougher to overeat them. People say potatoes or yams make them fat. But it's all the sour cream, butter, and cheese you put on it. Oftentimes a carb food is a vehicle for more fat, sugar, and salt."
>>Go easy on dairy. Andrews says there aren't many benefits in adding dairy to the diet. "Most of the nutrients you get from dairy you can get easily from other sources," he says, "and a lot of it is really easy to overeat."

USE PROTEIN POWDERS. They're useful if you have trouble eating protein foods frequently, and much more convenient than cooking and lugging around chicken and beef regularly.
>>Splurge on real desserts. When people diet, they tend to embrace low-sugar ice cream and sugar-free pudding. Because these foods aren't as satisfying, people overindulge. In fact, Andrews points out that some of these "fake" desserts can end up being over 1,000 calories. Just eat a small cookie.

CHAPTER 16

NEXT LEVEL OF LEAN

GET HARDCORE IN YOUR FAT-BURNING EFFORTS WITH THESE SEVEN ADVANCED STRATEGIES

Fat loss has been a hot topic for about the last 50 years. The abs-obsessed public seems to have an insatiable appetite for all things ripped, and a slew of fat-loss information is proffered everywhere you look. Mainstream magazines tout diets that focus on whole grains while tabloids hawk the grapefruit-only meal plan that got some pop star down to 122 pounds (but still at 28% body fat).

If you're a regular *Muscle & Fitness* reader, most of that fat-loss info available for public consumption just isn't relevant to you: It's either way too basic or just plain ridiculous. When "toned" is too soft and "fit" is too flimsy, you need something that's more advanced. With your kind of training schedule and clean diet, you need a serious, hardcore fat-loss plan—something that can take you from "That guy is pretty fit" to "That guy is ripped!"

These tips can help. They're designed specifically for the seasoned, experienced lifter who never skips workouts and already eats a clean and conscientious diet but wants to take his leanness to another level.

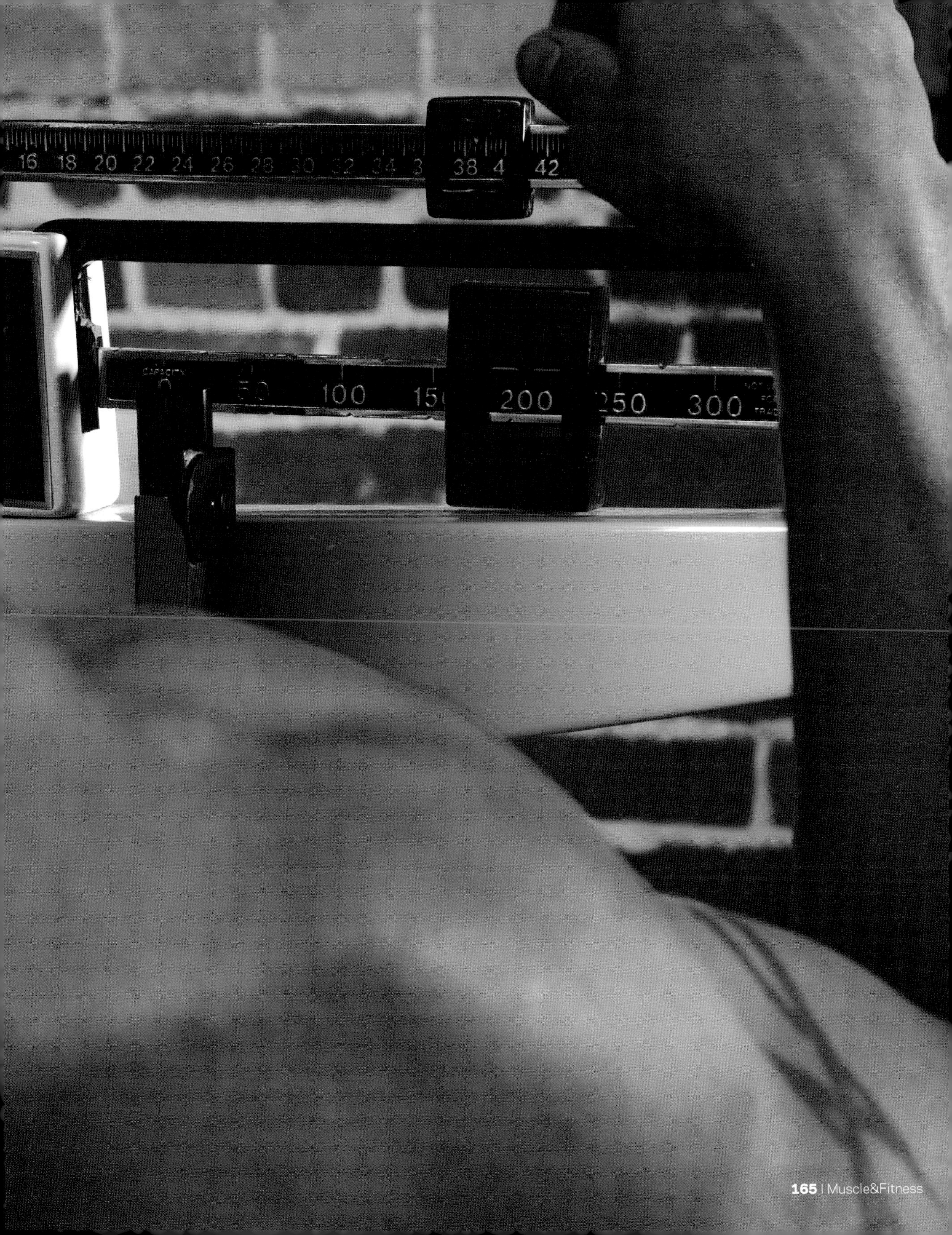
16 18 20 22 24 26 28 30 32 34 38 42
CAPACITY
0 50 100 200 250 300

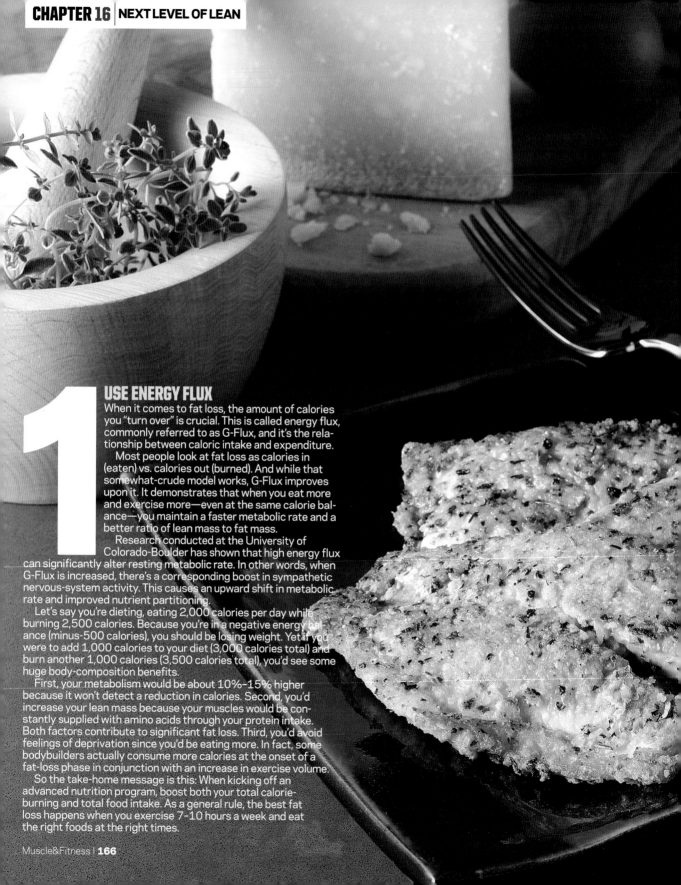

1 USE ENERGY FLUX

When it comes to fat loss, the amount of calories you "turn over" is crucial. This is called energy flux, commonly referred to as G-Flux, and it's the relationship between caloric intake and expenditure.

Most people look at fat loss as calories in (eaten) vs. calories out (burned). And while that somewhat-crude model works, G-Flux improves upon it. It demonstrates that when you eat more and exercise more—even at the same calorie balance—you maintain a faster metabolic rate and a better ratio of lean mass to fat mass.

Research conducted at the University of Colorado-Boulder has shown that high energy flux can significantly alter resting metabolic rate. In other words, when G-Flux is increased, there's a corresponding boost in sympathetic nervous-system activity. This causes an upward shift in metabolic rate and improved nutrient partitioning.

Let's say you're dieting, eating 2,000 calories per day while burning 2,500 calories. Because you're in a negative energy balance (minus-500 calories), you should be losing weight. Yet if you were to add 1,000 calories to your diet (3,000 calories total) and burn another 1,000 calories (3,500 calories total), you'd see some huge body-composition benefits.

First, your metabolism would be about 10%-15% higher because it won't detect a reduction in calories. Second, you'd increase your lean mass because your muscles would be constantly supplied with amino acids through your protein intake. Both factors contribute to significant fat loss. Third, you'd avoid feelings of deprivation since you'd be eating more. In fact, some bodybuilders actually consume more calories at the onset of a fat-loss phase in conjunction with an increase in exercise volume.

So the take-home message is this: When kicking off an advanced nutrition program, boost both your total calorie-burning and total food intake. As a general rule, the best fat loss happens when you exercise 7-10 hours a week and eat the right foods at the right times.

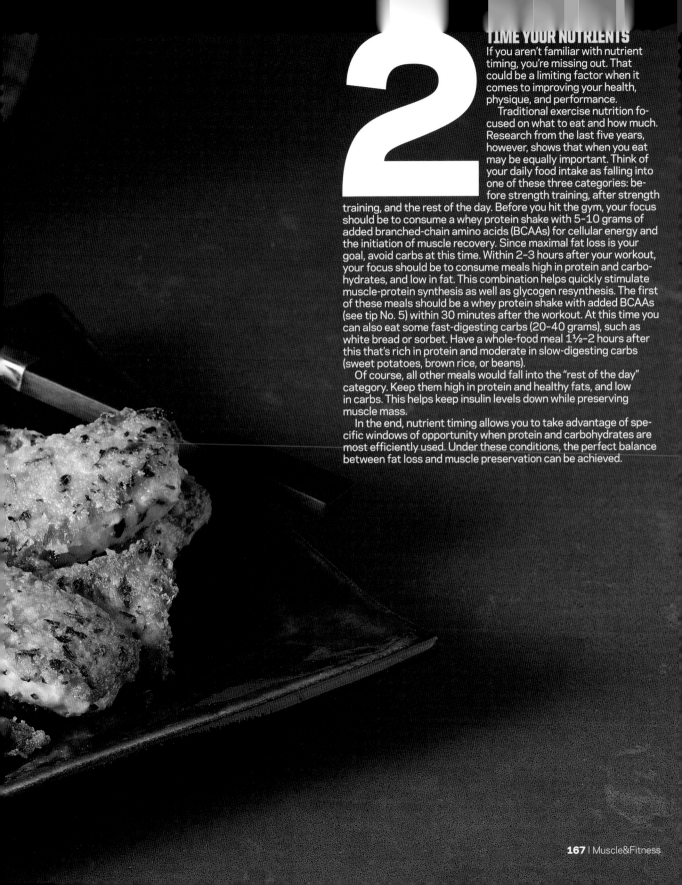

2 TIME YOUR NUTRIENTS

If you aren't familiar with nutrient timing, you're missing out. That could be a limiting factor when it comes to improving your health, physique, and performance.

Traditional exercise nutrition focused on what to eat and how much. Research from the last five years, however, shows that when you eat may be equally important. Think of your daily food intake as falling into one of these three categories: before strength training, after strength training, and the rest of the day. Before you hit the gym, your focus should be to consume a whey protein shake with 5–10 grams of added branched-chain amino acids (BCAAs) for cellular energy and the initiation of muscle recovery. Since maximal fat loss is your goal, avoid carbs at this time. Within 2–3 hours after your workout, your focus should be to consume meals high in protein and carbohydrates, and low in fat. This combination helps quickly stimulate muscle-protein synthesis as well as glycogen resynthesis. The first of these meals should be a whey protein shake with added BCAAs (see tip No. 5) within 30 minutes after the workout. At this time you can also eat some fast-digesting carbs (20–40 grams), such as white bread or sorbet. Have a whole-food meal 1½–2 hours after this that's rich in protein and moderate in slow-digesting carbs (sweet potatoes, brown rice, or beans).

Of course, all other meals would fall into the "rest of the day" category. Keep them high in protein and healthy fats, and low in carbs. This helps keep insulin levels down while preserving muscle mass.

In the end, nutrient timing allows you to take advantage of specific windows of opportunity when protein and carbohydrates are most efficiently used. Under these conditions, the perfect balance between fat loss and muscle preservation can be achieved.

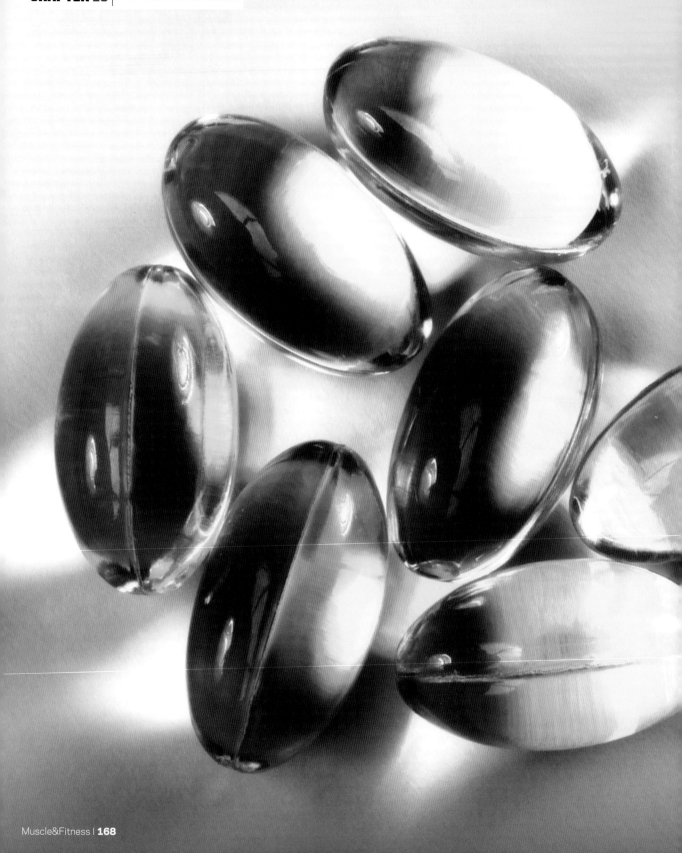

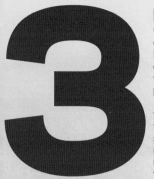

3

BURN FAT WITH FISH OIL

Omega-3 fats such as flax oil and fish oil were once the exclusive domain of health nuts and gym rats. Yet in the last few years the mainstream consumer has begun to embrace their use. Unfortunately, in the process the weightlifting community seems to have forgotten how powerful these dietary fats are.

Current research may revive our interest in omega-3 fats, especially the EPA- and DHA-rich fish oil. Research from the University of Western Ontario in Canada has shown that supplementing with fish oil can boost resting metabolic rate by 300–400 calories per day. In addition, new research indicates that fish oil can improve carb tolerance and decrease inflammation, and it has been found to provide a host of benefits across the health and wellness spectrum.

Be aware, however, that the minimum dosages recommended by most manufacturers are too low to offer the physique benefits most hard-training guys are looking for. For maximum benefit, start off a fat-loss program by taking about 1 gram of fish oil per percent body fat, up to a maximum of 30 grams. So if your body fat is 15%, you'd take 15 grams of fish oil. After about four weeks, drop the dose to about 0.5 gram per percent body fat. If you don't have a precise take on your body fat percentage, go with 12–15 grams for the first four weeks and then cut it in half to 6–7 grams after that.

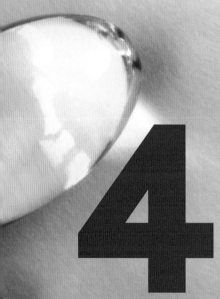

4

CYCLE YOUR CALORIES

As your diet progresses and your calories drop, your exercise volume will have to increase. This creates a highly negative energy balance that'll eventually cause a metabolic slowdown. But that's not all; sex hormone and anabolic hormone output will also diminish. This means your fat-loss progress will drop while muscle begins to waste away.

To prevent this results-squashing sequence of events, start cycling your calories in the later stages of a fat-loss program, at about the 8-10-week mark. But instead of just cycling calories, cycle your macronutrients as well. One great way to do this is to devise four different menu plans (see accompanying sidebar). By varying your amounts of calories, carbs, and fats, you prevent falling into "starvation mode" and make your fat loss more continuous. In addition, a varied diet like this one is psychologically easier to follow.

MENU 1:
Low calories, lower carbs, low fat
MONDAY, TUESDAY, FRIDAY, SATURDAY
-9 calories per pound of body weight
-50–70g carbs/day
-30–60g fat/day
-*Protein makes up the rest of your calories.*

MENU 2:
Moderate calories, higher carbs, low fat
THURSDAY
-11 calories per pound of body weight
-100–140g carbs/day
-30–60g fat/day
-*Protein makes up the rest of your calories.*

MENU 3:
High calories, high carbs, high fat
SUNDAY
-13 calories per pound of body weight
-200–280g carbs/day
-60–120g fat/day
-*Protein makes up the rest of your calories.*

MENU 4:
High calories, low carbs, high fat
WEDNESDAY
-13 calories per pound of body weight
-30–50g carbs/day
-60–120g fat/day
-*Protein makes up the rest of your calories.*

5

BCAAs & CREATINE

Many dieters find that their muscle mass really starts to drop off as a diet continues. To combat this, try supplementing with BCAAs and creatine. The BCAAs, especially leucine, have powerful anti-catabolic effects that can help stimulate protein synthesis and a positive protein balance. Creatine can assist in the preservation of muscle-cell volume as well as performance during a low-calorie phase. Both can also aid fat loss. Together, these supplements can help prevent muscle loss during a strict diet.

The best strategy is to take 5–10 grams of BCAAs with breakfast, your pre- and post-workout shakes, and a meal late in the day. Take 2–5 grams of creatine with your pre- and post-workout shakes. On rest days, take creatine with BCAAs at breakfast.

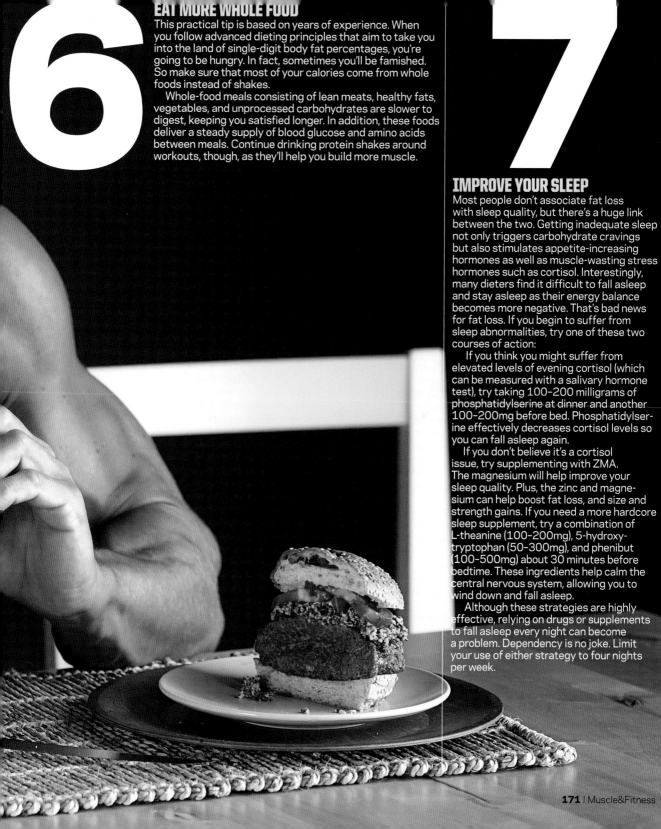

6

EAT MORE WHOLE FOOD

This practical tip is based on years of experience. When you follow advanced dieting principles that aim to take you into the land of single-digit body fat percentages, you're going to be hungry. In fact, sometimes you'll be famished. So make sure that most of your calories come from whole foods instead of shakes.

Whole-food meals consisting of lean meats, healthy fats, vegetables, and unprocessed carbohydrates are slower to digest, keeping you satisfied longer. In addition, these foods deliver a steady supply of blood glucose and amino acids between meals. Continue drinking protein shakes around workouts, though, as they'll help you build more muscle.

7

IMPROVE YOUR SLEEP

Most people don't associate fat loss with sleep quality, but there's a huge link between the two. Getting inadequate sleep not only triggers carbohydrate cravings but also stimulates appetite-increasing hormones as well as muscle-wasting stress hormones such as cortisol. Interestingly, many dieters find it difficult to fall asleep and stay asleep as their energy balance becomes more negative. That's bad news for fat loss. If you begin to suffer from sleep abnormalities, try one of these two courses of action:

If you think you might suffer from elevated levels of evening cortisol (which can be measured with a salivary hormone test), try taking 100–200 milligrams of phosphatidylserine at dinner and another 100–200mg before bed. Phosphatidylserine effectively decreases cortisol levels so you can fall asleep again.

If you don't believe it's a cortisol issue, try supplementing with ZMA. The magnesium will help improve your sleep quality. Plus, the zinc and magnesium can help boost fat loss, and size and strength gains. If you need a more hardcore sleep supplement, try a combination of L-theanine (100–200mg), 5-hydroxytryptophan (50–300mg), and phenibut (100–500mg) about 30 minutes before bedtime. These ingredients help calm the central nervous system, allowing you to wind down and fall asleep.

Although these strategies are highly effective, relying on drugs or supplements to fall asleep every night can become a problem. Dependency is no joke. Limit your use of either strategy to four nights per week.

TRACK YOUR PROGRESS

KEEPING A JOURNAL OF YOUR TRAINING AND DIET WILL HELP YOU STAY ON TRACK. HERE ARE THREE BLANK JOURNAL PAGES YOU CAN PHOTOCOPY TO GET YOU STARTED.

DATE _____

WEIGHT TRAINING SESSION

WARMUP	EXERCISE	DURATION

BODY PART	EXERCISE	SET 1 REPS	WT	SET 2 REPS	WT	SET 3 REPS	WT	SET 4 REPS	WT

CARDIO TRAINING SESSION

EXERCISE	NOTES
DURATION	

NUTRITION JOURNAL

MEAL 1	CAL	PROTEIN	CARBS	FAT	MEAL 4	CAL	PROTEIN	CARBS	FAT

MEAL 2	CAL	PROTEIN	CARBS	FAT	MEAL 5	CAL	PROTEIN	CARBS	FAT

MEAL 3	CAL	PROTEIN	CARBS	FAT	MEAL 6	CAL	PROTEIN	CARBS	FAT

DAILY TOTALS	CALORIES:	PROTEIN:	CARBS:	FAT:

EXERCISE LOG

DATE _____

WEIGHT TRAINING SESSION

WARMUP	EXERCISE	DURATION

BODY PART	EXERCISE	SET 1 REPS	WT	SET 2 REPS	WT	SET 3 REPS	WT	SET 4 REPS	WT

CARDIO TRAINING SESSION

EXERCISE	NOTES
DURATION	

NUTRITION JOURNAL

MEAL 1	CAL	PROTEIN	CARBS	FAT	MEAL 4	CAL	PROTEIN	CARBS	FAT

MEAL 2	CAL	PROTEIN	CARBS	FAT	MEAL 5	CAL	PROTEIN	CARBS	FAT

MEAL 3	CAL	PROTEIN	CARBS	FAT	MEAL 6	CAL	PROTEIN	CARBS	FAT

DAILY TOTALS	CALORIES:	PROTEIN:	CARBS:	FAT:

DATE _____

WEIGHT TRAINING SESSION

WARMUP	EXERCISE	DURATION

BODY PART	EXERCISE	SET 1 REPS	WT	SET 2 REPS	WT	SET 3 REPS	WT	SET 4 REPS	WT

CARDIO TRAINING SESSION

EXERCISE	NOTES
DURATION	

NUTRITION JOURNAL

MEAL 1	CAL	PROTEIN	CARBS	FAT	MEAL 4	CAL	PROTEIN	CARBS	FAT
MEAL 2	CAL	PROTEIN	CARBS	FAT	**MEAL 5**	CAL	PROTEIN	CARBS	FAT
MEAL 3	CAL	PROTEIN	CARBS	FAT	**MEAL 6**	CAL	PROTEIN	CARBS	FAT
DAILY TOTALS	CALORIES:		PROTEIN:		CARBS:		FAT:		